I0092810

AGING

A Healthy Meaningful Journey
(Health span matching life span)

Dr. Richard Ng, DO

ISBN 978-1-956001-35-8 (paperback)
ISBN 978-1-956001-36-5 (eBook)

Copyright © 2021 by Dr. Richard Ng, DO

All rights reserved. No part of this publication may be reproduced, distributed, or transmitted in any form or by any means, including photocopying, recording, or other electronic or mechanical methods without the prior written permission of the publisher.

Printed in the United States of America

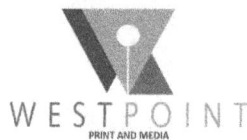

WEST POINT
PRINT AND MEDIA

In memory of my dear parents.
Passed on and buried in Elmhurst, Illinois, USA

CONTENTS

Foreword..vii

Chapter 1:   Aging and cardiovascular diseases 1

Chapter 2:   Aging and Cancers 13

Chapter 3:   Aging and the Mind..37

Chapter 4:   Aging and Sex 54

Chapter 5:   Aging : Looking Healthy and Youthful............................65

Chapter 6:   Aging and Longevity 83

Chapter 7:   Aging and Supplements..105

Chapter 8:   Aging and Constipation 142

Chapter 9:   Aging and Frailty..147

Chapter 10: Aging and Walking..156

Chapter 11: Spirituality and Faith...166

Chapter 12: Epilogue and Happy Aging 174

FOREWORD

Well, we know that people are living longer, but that does not necessarily mean that they are living healthier. The increase in our aging population presents some public health challenges that we need to prepare for.

The world's older population continues to grow at an unprecedented rate. Today, almost 9 percent of people worldwide (625 million) are aged 65 and over. This percentage is projected to jump to nearly 17 percent of the world's population by 2050 (1.6 billion approximately). In the U.S., the 65- and—over population is projected to nearly double over the next three decades, from the current 48 million to 88 million by 2050.

What is aging? Ageing (British English) or aging (American English) is the process of becoming older. In the narrow sense, the term refers to biological aging of human beings, animals and other organisms. In the broader sense, aging can refer to single cells within an organism (cellular aging) or to the population (population aging).

Nature or nurture?

There are several theories about aging: the aging-clock theory, the genetic theory, the immunological theory, and the free-radical theory. The free-radical theory is the most commonly held theory at the present time; it is based on the fact that on-going chemical reactions of the cells produce free radicals. In the presence of oxygen, these free radicals, under oxidative stress, cause the cells of the body to break down. As time goes on, more cells die or lose the ability to function, and the body eventually ceases to function as a whole. Antioxidants can help to normalize damage by the free radical actions that contribute to the problems of aging.

Aging is a multi-faceted process in which bodily structures and functions undergo a negative deviation from the optimum—growing old. The time of your life when age-related changes appear depends on a variety of factors, including :

- Genetics
- Diet
- Culture
- Activity levels
- Environmental exposure
- Mental health

Let us briefly look at the bodily functions and structures that are most often affected by age:

Hearing—this auditory function declines with age and you will find it harder and harder to hear, especially in relation to the highest-pitched tones. If this impairment is not corrected, it can have significant adverse impact on one's mental health including cognition.

Fat increase—the proportion of fat to muscle may increase by as much as 30 percent. Typically, the total padding of body fat directly under the skin thins out and accumulates around the abdominal area. The ability to excrete is reduced and therefore the storage of fats increase, including cholesterol and fat-soluble nutrients.

Decrease of body water—with the decreasing concentration of body water, there is a decrease of the absorption of water-soluble nutrients. Also, there is less saliva and other lubricating fluids. Most of us tend to take water for granted because it is so freely and readily available almost everywhere. Ironically, many of us are not drinking enough water, and chronic dehydration is actually quite common. Adequate concentration of water in the body is very important for our physical and mental health.

To make matter worse, as we get older, we lose the sharpness, acuity and precision of our senses including hearing, vision, taste, smell and thirst. Due to the gradual loss of the sense of thirst, the elderly are facing an increased risk of dehydration, especially at the cellular levels. Studies by Phillips and Associates have shown that after 24 hours of water deprivation, the elderly participants still do not realize or recognize that they are thirsty. Other studies published in the Lancet have supported the conclusion that the thirst mechanism is gradually lost in the elderly with aging.

Liver—it weighs about three and a half pounds, serving as an indispensable processing warehouse for the body. Aging has been shown to not only heighten vulnerability to acute liver injury but also increase susceptibility of the fibrotic responses. Moreover, aging increases the risk of various liver diseases including non-alcoholic fatty liver disease (NAFLD), alcoholic liver disease for drinkers and hepatitis; aging unfortunately implies poor prognosis for liver transplantation. The ability of the liver to metabolize many substances decreases with aging. Thus, some drugs are not inactivated as quickly and efficiently in older people as they are in younger people. In general, treatment of older people with liver diseases may require different and/or longer intervention.

The kidneys—they are two bean-shaped organs found on the right and left in the retroperitoneal space of the body; normally, they are about 12 to 13 centimeters in length in adult humans. Kidney function declines naturally with age, even if a person is in good health. With aging, the amount of kidney tissues decreases, and the number of filtering units, called nephrons, diminishes, thus decreasing their capacity to filter wastes from the blood and to remove extra fluid from the body. With aging, the blood vessels supplying the kidneys can become hardened, causing kidneys to filter blood more slowly

The loss of kidney function happens to everyone; it is a matter of the extent of loss with variations as to how quickly this occurs.

Decrease in digestion—The digestive system includes the mouth, esophagus, stomach, pancreas, liver and gall bladder, small and large intestines, and the rectum. As you age, chewing can become more difficult, you may chew more slowly, and you may not chew your food as efficiently, especially if you have dentures or poor dentition. When you swallow larger pieces of food, it takes longer for it to make its way to your stomach because your esophagus does not contract as forcefully as it did when you were younger. With age, the stomach cannot accommodate as much food because of decreased elasticity, and the rate at which the stomach empties food into the small intestines also decreases. The muscles in the digestive tract become stiffer, weaker and less efficient. Constipation is a common problem among the elderly population.

Digestion is also more difficult due to a decrease in gastric acid production and reduced levels of digestive enzymes. Fortunately, your digestive system does not have to become a victim of age; it can often be protected with a healthy lifestyle including proper hydration, normal body weight, attention to portion sizes of food, sufficient amount of fiber in your diet and regular exercise.

Cardio-pulmonary system—aging brings an increased stiffness of the chest wall, diminished blood flow through the lungs, and a reduction in the strength of your heart beats. In fact, heart rate per minute generally declines with each year and can be estimated by subtracting your age from 220. These changes in your cardiovascular and respiratory systems lead to decreased oxygen and nutrients throughout the body.

People age 65 and older are much more likely than younger ones to suffer a heart attack, to have a stroke, or to develop heart failure. The most common age-related change is an increased stiffness of the arteries called arteriosclerosis, or hardening of the arteries. This causes elevated blood pressure, so hypertension is more common as we age. Advancing age also increases the risk for atherosclerosis with plaque buildup inside the arterial walls; overtime, this hardens and narrows the arteries, which reduce the flow of oxygen-rich blood to the organs and tissues of the body. Long-standing hypertension is the main cause of increased heart size, cardiomegaly, which can increase the risk of atrial fibrillation, a common cardiac problem in the geriatric group.

Age-related changes in the electrical system of the heart can lead to arrhythmia—a rapid, slowed or irregular heartbeat. Moreover, the chambers of the heart may increase in size with thickening of the walls; thus, the amount of blood that a heart chamber can hold can decrease despite the increased overall size of the heart.

Effects of aging on the respiratory system include a smaller rib-cage. As the muscles between the ribs become weaker, the rib-cage contracts around the lungs can make breathing more difficult when one becomes older, especially with exertion in a sedentary lifestyle. Therefore, regular exercise can increase blood flow, which in turn strengthens the lungs and ensures better exchange of air.

A decrease in bone strength and density—your bones are bustling with activities, being constantly remodeled; they are in a continuous cycle of destruction and renewal until the day you die. The problem is, as time passes you lose more bone than you make. As a result, bones become thinner and more susceptible to fracture. As this process accelerates after age 50, osteoporosis becomes more common. Osteoporosis is a condition of progressive bone loss that is painful, debilitating, disfiguring with loss of height and increased risk of fractures. Unfortunately, the rate of bone loss accelerates by about 10 folds after menopause for women.

The aging process can cause loss of calcium and other minerals in the bones; the overall age-related bone changes have a direct adverse effect on joint mobility. Joint movements become stiffer and less flexible because the amount of synovial fluid inside the synovial joints decreases and the cartilages become thinner. Aging also causes the ligaments of joints to shorten, losing some flexibility; the subchondral bone (the layer directly below the articular cartilage) also suffers a reduction in thickness and density.

Loss of muscle strength and coordination—aging causes reduction in protein formation leading to shrinkage in muscle mass and decreased bone formation, resulting in gradual loss of mobility, agility, and flexibility.

Our muscles provide the force and strength to move the body. Coordination is directed by the brain, but is affected by changes in the muscles and joints. Aging muscles tend to shrink with smaller mass due to the reduction in the number and size of muscle fibers. The water content of tendons that attach muscles to bones also decrease with age.

With decreasing muscle strength, it becomes more difficult to accomplish routine activities such as opening a jar or bottle, or turning the key of a lock. Immobility such as being bed-ridden and malnutrition can accelerate the loss of muscle mass in a short time, even though the loss of muscle mass is a normal condition when getting older. The elderly segment of our population are very prone and susceptible to this, and can lead to frailty.

Olfactory functions—there is a decrease in the sensations of taste and smell as you get older, besides the age-related hearing impairment already mentioned. Thus, older people tend to be less stimulated by food than the young, leading to some change or loss of appetite which is common in the elderly.

Other sensations such as pain, touch and temperature are affected by aging due to gradual loss of skin receptors.

There is a decline in the production of sexual hormones, both testosterone and estrogen, leading to diminished sexual functioning. Other hormone levels are also decreased, especially the thyroid hormones.

The loss of sex hormones in aging may be responsible for some muscle loss, muscle weakness, and decreased functional performance. The ovaries and testes have two primary functions: they produce the reproductive cells (ova and sperm), and they produce the sex hormones that control the secondary sex characteristics such as breasts and facial hair. For men, with the decline of testosterone, he may hind himself thinking about sex less often, his penile erections may not be as robust, and he may not get turned on as easily as he did when he was younger.

Decreased functioning of the nervous system—your nerve impulses are not transmitted as efficiently, reflexes are not as sharp, and memory and learning are diminished. It might take longer to learn new things or remember familiar words or names.

With aging, the brain and spinal cord lose nerve cells (neurons) and weight (atrophy or cerebral thinning). The neurons may pass messages more slowly than in the past. Toxic wastes can collect in the brain tissue as neurons break down and this can cause abnormal changes in the brain called plaques and tangles. The fatty myelin that wraps around the axons deteriorates and the number of connections or synapses between neurons may drop, affecting learning and memory.

The function of the automatic nervous system (ANS) also decline with aging, as shown by many studies. It is undeniable that the human brain does deteriorate with age, but many studies have shown neuro-protection with some strategies and activities.

Declining visual function—your vision changes with your age with the development of cataracts and age-related macular degeneration resulting in poor visual acuity. Many older people have presbyopia with the inability to focus or accommodate due to inflexible lenses of the eyes. There is also a gradual loss of peripheral vision, atrophy of lacrimal glands, and difficulty in discriminating certain colors.

The integumentary system (skin)—this is the largest organ of the body, and in which changes associated with aging are most visible. The glandular secretions decrease, resulting in dry skin and increased susceptibility to infections. The reduction in sweat production, the loss of subcutaneous, adipose tissue, especially in the extremities, and poor skin circulation all affect thermoregulation.

The dermis, which is responsible for the elasticity and resilience of the skin, exhibits a reduced ability to regenerate, leading to slower wound healing. The hypodermis, with its fat stores, loses its accessory structures along with reduced fat storage. These age-related changes contribute to the thinning and sagging of skin; the skin on the face and hands, generally, starts to show the first sign of aging.

Your ability to produce vitamin D from sunlight when your skin is exposed is also compromised.

All these age-related physical and physiological changes just described should not be looked at as death sentences. You can't change the genes you inherited, but you can avoid bad habits and bad foods that contribute to your health problems.

Human beings reach a peak of growth and development around the time of their mid-20s. Aging is among the biggest known risk factors for most human diseases: of the roughly 150,000 people who die every day across the globe, about two thirds die from age-related causes.

CHAPTER ONE

Aging and cardiovascular diseases

With much of the medical advances we have made so far in the twenty-first century, heart disease is still the leading cause of death in the United States. This trend and phenomenon are multi-factorial, but we can all agree that our lifestyle, behavior and diet together play a major role in this disturbing statistics.

As we get older, we face increasing risk of hypertension, stroke, heart attack, and other cardiovascular diseases.

High blood pressure is a common condition that will catch up with most people who live into older age. Blood pressure is the force of blood pressing against the walls of the arteries. Hypertension is sometimes called a silent killer because it may have no obvious symptoms for years. In fact, many people, at least over 20 percent of our population, with this condition do not know they have high blood pressure. In most cases, the underlying causes of high blood pressure are unknown. Overtime, it can quietly damage the heart, lungs, blood vessels, brain and kidneys.

Sodium, a major component of common salt, can raise the blood pressure by causing the body to retain fluid, which leads to greater burden on the heart. The American Heart Association recommends eating less than 1500mg of Sodium per day. Processed foods including canned soup and lunch meats make up the majority of our sodium intake.

Being overweight places a strain on the heart and increases your risk of hypertension, among many other health problems your excess body weight can create. Obesity and overweight have become a major public health problem, having reached an epidemic proportion. Its negative and serious impact on heart health is undeniable.

Drinking too much alcohol can increase your blood pressure. Guidelines from the American Heart Association state that you should limit the amount no more than two drinks a day for men, or one drink a day for women. One drink is defined as one 12-ounce beer, 4 ounces of wine and one ounce of 100-proof spirits. It is best not to drink alcohol at all due to its many harmful effects on the body, especially of chronic alcoholics.

Studies have not shown any link between caffeine (coffee) and development of hypertension. You can safely drink one or two cups of coffee a day, according to the American Heart Association, as long as you are careful with the sugar and creamer. It is best to enjoy your coffee black without sugar and cream. Being the most prevalent and common beverage in the U.S. today, coffee beans are an excellent source of antioxidants. Coffee beans also contain many vitamins and minerals, such as riboflavin, pantothenic acid, niacin, thiamine, folic acid, zinc, potassium, manganese and magnesium.

Cigarettes contain nicotine which narrows the blood vessels and thus raises the cardiac work load, leading to elevated blood pressure. Another complication is the carbon monoxide with smoking; it takes the place of oxygen in your blood. This puts a burden on your heart because the heart has to work harder to circulate sufficient oxygen needed by the tissues, eventually raising your blood pressure.

Do yourself a big favor and quit smoking cigarettes, including avoidance of second-hand smoking.

Most people are familiar with the heightened risk of lung cancer associated with cigarette smoking, but unaware of, ignoring, or not realizing the multiple serious health consequences of smoking. It tends to accelerate the aging processes of the body; smokers are more likely to develop facial wrinkles and a haggard look. Cigarette contains hundreds of harmful chemicals, besides nicotine. The air pollutants in the smoke and the toxic chemicals in the cigarette greatly increase the oxidative activities throughout the body, with the elevated levels of free radicals overwhelming and tilting the body's equilibrium. The hundreds of free radicals in a single puff of cigarette smoke also trigger inflammatory cells, adding more toxins and stress to the body including the heart.

Excessive sugar intake increases insulin in the blood stream. Chronic high insulin levels cause tense arterial walls, leading to high blood pressure. It is scary to know that sugar is one of the biggest heart-damaging culprits in our modern society, and many people are not aware of it or they are subconsciously denying it.

The average American consumes about 80 pounds of added sugar annually, or more than 23 teaspoons of added sugar daily. Poor control of blood sugar is the hallmark of diabetes mellitus. Excess glucose reacts with proteins to form Advanced Glycation End-products (AGEs), blocking normal functioning and altering the structures of proteins. The AGEs tend to become sticky when there is too much sugar in the blood, adversely affecting different organs of the body, including the heart, kidneys and the brain.

Certain medications including over the counter cold and flu medicines contain decongestants that can cause blood pressure to rise. Others include non-steroidal anti-inflammatory drugs, like ibuprofen and naproxen for pain relief OTC, steroids, diet pills, birth control pills, and some antidepressants. So, consult your physicians about this.

Exercise can help decrease your blood pressure. You should get about 150 minutes of moderate-intensity activity every week, such as swimming, brisk walking, gardening and biking. The innumerable benefits of exercise and walking on cardiovascular, physical and mental health are undisputable. Our modern, digital world tends to encourage a sedentary lifestyle, with many serious health consequences, especially the cardiopulmonary system.

An inactive lifestyle will weaken and stiffen the musculoskeletal systems; your circulatory system will slow down with stasis. Your heart and lungs will have diminished functional capacities, delivery less nutrients and oxygen to different organs and tissues of the body with the heart and brain being the most critical ones.

Meditation, yoga, tai chi and other relaxation techniques can reduce your stress and blood pressure levels, giving you a sense of comfort and peace. Elevated levels of stress and feelings of sadness can be detrimental to cardiac health.

Getting seven to eight hours of sleep a night is important for heart health and our general well-being. Poor sleep or sleep deprivation is linked to higher blood pressure, which is a risk factor for heart disease. We all need adequate quality sleep with " down time " necessary to eliminate metabolic wastes optimally. Older people in general are light sleepers because they spend less time in the deep stages of sleep cycle.

Have a gratitude journal—studies have shown that expressing gratitude is positive for your heart health with lower levels of inflammatory bio-markers.

Always find something to laugh about—laughter is indeed the best medicine—it lowers your stress, dilates the arteries and keeps the blood pressure down.

Drinking enough water—the amount should be half of your body weight in ounces. For example, if you weigh 150 pounds, you should drink at least 75 ounces of water a day. Of course, allow more with certain activities. Dehydration can lead to increased hematocrit and blood viscosity, both of which have been associated with cardiovascular events.

Many of us tend to take water for granted and chronic dehydration is quite common. The human body has not stored water to draw from in the case of dehydration; that is why we must drink water regularly and throughout the day, unless you have a medical need for fluid restriction under the advice of your physician.

Stroke is the third leading cause of death in the United States. It is a rather common and devastating event among the senior population, which often results in death or significant loss of independence with tremendous human and financial costs.

Medically, it is also known as cerebrovascular accident (CVA), brain attack or cerebrovascular insult. It occurs when poor blood flow to the brain results in cell death. There are two main types of stroke: ischemic due to poor or lack of blood flow, and hemorrhagic due to bleeding.

Without awareness with public education, lifestyle changes and healthy eating, the burden of stroke, both economically and socially will continue to grow, contributing to the already high health care costs. We have sufficient scientific evidence that dietary habits, not only influence the prevalence of stroke, but also its course and outcome once it has occurred.

There are many risk factors for stroke, and the major ones include high blood pressure, high lipid levels, diabetes, excess body weight and heart disease. According to the Center for Disease Control and Prevention, cigarette smoking is, in particular, a high risk for stroke.

Control your diabetes—If you are diabetic, you need to cut back on drinks and foods with added sugar and maintain a healthy, balanced diet. People with diabetes suffer higher incidence of heart disease, stroke and kidney disease unfortunately; it is the nature of the beast and you must do your best to tame it in order to have a longer, healthy and meaningful life.

There are things you can do to prevent or lower your risk for a stroke:

- Smoking cessation
- Avoiding excess sugar
- Limiting alcohol consumption
- Avoiding trans and saturated fats
- Be physically active and exercise regularly.
- Avoiding excessive salt
- Eating more fish with heart-healthy omega-3 fatty acids
- Eating more fruits and vegetables
- Eating more whole grain high-fiber foods
- Cooking more at home
- Consult your physician about staring the low-dose aspirin regimen

Many of us are familiar with the two frightful words, heart attack, and older people are at increased risk for myocardial infarction. The most common symptom is chest pain when blood flow to the heart is compromised, blocked or decreased. Heart attack occurs when the blood flow to a part of the heart stops, causing damage to the heart muscle. Other symptoms include vague chest discomfort, pain traveling to the shoulder, upper arm, back, neck or jaw. It may be disguised as a heart burn sometimes.

In the U.S., more than 170,000 men and women died from a heart attack annually. The international research team created the Fatty acids and Outcomes Research Consortium (FORCE) and found common foods like salmon, mackerel, walnuts, pecans and hazelnuts may be a way to eat your way to a higher rate of survival from a heart attack, according to the Journal of American Medical Association. These findings put doubt to rest about the positive effects that omega-3 fatty acids can have on a person's heart.

The heart, normally, continues to pump enough blood to supply all parts of the body. However, an older heart may not be able to pump blood as well when you make it work harder. Here are some of the things that make your heart work harder:

- Certain medications
- Emotional stress
- Physical exertion
- Illness
- Fever
- Infections
- Injuries
- Anemia
- Malnutrition
- Blood loss from the gastrointestinal tract, acute or chronic
- Atherosclerosis

The American Heart Association suggests a diet rich in fruits and vegetables, whole grains, low-fat dairy products, lean poultry, fish and nuts. According to one study, strawberries and blueberries can increase blood flow in your heart and may decrease the likelihood of a heart attack. In a 2014 Framingham Heart Study report, lack of sufficient magnesium in the diet was determined to be a risk factor for cardiovascular disease. Magnesium was found to help prevent calcification of the coronary arteries in the study.

From a nutritional stand point, a healthy diet for your cardiovascular system should include foods that can improve blood flow, fight plaque buildup, lower the bad cholesterol in the blood, stabilize the blood sugar, and reduce inflammation in your arteries.

The following is a list of heart-healthy foods which are common and not difficult to incorporate into your daily diet:

- Dark chocolate—it contains flavonoids, the antioxidants that help lower LDL levels. Just make sure to consume in moderation, as it is also high in saturated fat and sugar.
- Avocados—it contains oleic acid which decreases bad cholesterol in your blood stream.
- Red wine—it contains resveratrol, an antioxidant found in the skin of red grapes. It is known to decrease levels of LDL and the risk of blood clots. But be sure to follow the recommended guidelines and not overdo it.
- Green/black tea—it contains powerful antioxidants that may decrease your LDL levels.
- Fish—their omega-3 fatty acids can reduce the stickiness of blood platelets, making them less likely to form clots, thus lessening the risk for strokes. The omega-3 fatty acids can also reduce inflammation of arterial walls and lower triglyceride levels.
- Whole grains—these include brown rice, oatmeal, barley and quinoa. They contain soluble fiber which helps remove cholesterol from the body and prevents plaques from forming in the arteries.
- Beans and legumes—they are high in protein, fiber, B vitamins, iron, potassium and other minerals while being low in fat. Their phytochemicals including isoflavones, are protective against heart disease. Their soluble fiber can reduce LDL cholesterol by as much as 10%, according to some studies.
- Fruits like apples, oranges and lemons have a lot of pectin, which is a type of fiber capable of reducing your cholesterol.

- Asparagus—it is a natural diuretic which helps your body get rid of excess fluid and salt, reducing the risk for high blood pressure.
- Bananas—they contain potassium which helps counter the adverse effects of sodium to regulate your blood pressure.
- Garlic—it is known to lower blood pressure and reduce atherosclerosis.
- Onions—they may inhibit the activation of platelets, preventing clogging of arteries.
- Tomatoes—they contain lycopene which helps dilate the blood vessels and maintain healthy blood flow.
- Grapes—besides their beneficial resveratrol found in their red wine, they also contain quercetin, a plant pigment that helps regulate blood cholesterol and reduce clot-forming platelets.
- Berries—these include blueberries, strawberries, raspberries and blackberries. They have strong anti-inflammatory properties to help lower blood pressure and raise the levels of good cholesterol (HDL).
- Cinnamon—it is a spice obtained from the inner bark of trees in the genus Cinnamomum. It has, among its multiple health benefits, anti-inflammatory properties which can protect against heart disease. It can help decrease cholesterol levels, keep the blood vessels clean and healthy. It contains coumarin, which prevents your blood from getting too thick and ensure blood to flow freely for oxygenation of the organs in your body.
- Nuts—these include walnuts, pistachios and almonds. They are packed with antioxidants and omega-3 fatty acids that can reduce the risk of heart disease. The most comprehensive review of clinical trials on nut consumption in relation to cardiovascular disease showed consuming just one ounce of

walnuts five times a week—about a handful each time—can slash heart disease risk by as much as 40 percent. Besides being one of the best dietary sources of polyunsaturated fats, walnuts have high amounts of copper, biotin, magnesium and molybdenum which are all essential for the health of your body.

- Grapefruits—in an Israeli study of men and women who had bypass surgeries and whose cholesterol levels were not responding to statin medications, those who ate a red grapefruit a day for a period of 30 days lowered their total cholesterol by more than 15%, their LDL cholesterol by more than 20%, and their triglycerides by more than 17%.

A word of caution: grapefruits can have dangerous interactions with certain medications including heart medicines; so check with your doctor before adding them to your diet. Grapefruit and juice contain natural chemical called furanocoumarin which can interfere with your liver metabolizing certain allergy medications such as Allegra and Claritin, resulting in elevated blood levels of the drugs. Grapefruit may interact with medications used to treat erectile dysfunction such as Viagra, Cialis and Levitra. It may prolong erection, causing a painful and potentially damaging side effect known as priapism. Many people take statin prescription medications to lower their cholesterol; they must be careful because grapefruit can cause a buildup of the medicines in the blood stream resulting in potentially dangerous side effects.

- Celery—it is a good source of potassium, a mineral that aids muscle function and offsets some of the sodium's damaging effects on blood pressure.
- Mushrooms—these fungi are one of the best plant-based source of niacin, a vitamin that can help reduce the risk of

heart disease and atherosclerosis. Being a vasodilator, Niacin improves blood flow to different tissues of the body.

- Potatoes—a staple part of the diet for most people. They are high in both potassium and magnesium, which are important to help lower your blood pressure.
- Sunflower seeds—they are a wonderful source of all kinds of nutrients and minerals. In this instance, their magnesium content plays an important part in reducing your blood pressure.
- Leafy green vegetables—like kale and spinach, they are high in potassium, which helps regulate the balance between potassium and sodium for better blood pressure.
- Skimmed milk—milk is good for us due to calcium, but whole fat milk is not so healthy due to its high fat content. Skimmed milk is beneficial to those people that have high blood pressure due to calcium, which is effective in reducing the blood pressure.

CHAPTER TWO

Aging and Cancers

Advancing age is the most important risk factor for cancer overall, and for many individual cancer types. According to the most recent statistical data from the National Cancer Institute's Surveillance, Epidemiology, and End Results program, the median age of a cancer diagnosis is 66 years. This means that half of cancer cases occur in people below this age and half in people above this age. At least 25 percent of all new cancer cases are diagnosed in people aged 65 to 74.

Cancer is a frightful, unpleasant word, and most of the people do not like to hear, talk or think about it. When I was a medical student in Chicago, I found it rather difficult, uneasy and sad to have to inform my patients and their family of the diagnosis of cancer. It is non-discriminatory, meaning that it can happen to anyone regardless of sex, race, ethnicity, skin color and wealth (poor or rich). It can start almost anywhere in the human body.

Cancer is the name given to a collection of related diseases. Cancer is a genetic disease—that is, it is caused by changes to genes that control the way our cells function, especially how they grow and divide. Cancer cells differ from normal cells in many ways that allow them to grow out of control and become invasive.

U.S. has the seventh highest cancer rate in the world. About 300 of every 100,000 Americans develop cancers each year. These disturbing and shocking statistics were compiled by the American Institute of Cancer Research in Washington, D.C. For the most, development of cancer is a gradual process overtime, years or even decades, before causing symptoms to appear. This " slowness " of cancer development essentially gives us a golden opportunity to intervene and to block the evolution of a transformed cell into a mature cancer cell.

Essentially, most cancers, if not all, have three stages of development: initiation, promotion and progression. Initiation is actually a latency period, during which the first mutation appears in the cellular DNA. At this stage, the initiated cells have the potential to form tumors; if exposure to toxic or harmful agents continues, the cells can be promoted to become cancerous. Certain micro-nutrients or molecules in foods have the property of maintaining the initiated cells and potential tumors in a latent state and thus can prevent cancer from developing.

At the Promotion stage, this is the phase with the best opportunity to intervene in the prevention of cancer development. Currently, the majority of cancer research is focused on efforts of modification and manipulation of this stage of Promotion, including lifestyle changes.

In the third stage of cancer development called Progression, the mutated, transformed cells gain independence and grow rapidly or slowly depending on the type of cancer. They can invade surrounding tissue and spread to other parts of the body called metastasis.

It is usually not possible to know exactly why and/or how one person develops cancer and another person does not. However, many researchers have shown that certain risk factors may increase a person's chance of developing cancer. Researchers also have found that certain factors are linked to a lower risk of cancer, called cancer-risk protective factors.

Many cancer risk factors and protective factors were identified in epidemiological studies, showing that people who develop cancer are more or less likely to behave in certain ways or to be exposed to certain substances than those who do not develop cancer. When many studies all point to a similar association between a potential risk factor and an increased risk of cancer and when a possible mechanism exists that could explain how the risk factor could cause cancer, scientists can be more confident about the relationship between the two.

The National Cancer Institute (NCI) published a list that includes the most-studied known or suspected risk factors for cancer. Although some of these risk factors can be avoided, others—such as growing older—cannot. Limiting your exposure to avoidable risk factors may decrease your risk of developing certain cancers.

Let us look at the list of cancer-causing risk factors:

- Your age
- Your family history
- Your health conditions
- Cancer-causing substances in the environment
- Chronic inflammation
- Diet
- Obesity

- Hormones
- Immunosuppression
- Infectious agents
- Radiation
- Sunlight
- Alcohol
- Tobacco

As you can see, many of the risk factors in the list can be changed, reduced or eliminated through lifestyle changes, a healthy, balanced diet and appropriate, regular physical activity. We are going to discuss about those risk factors that you can change and maximize the protective factors. Our high cancer ranking in the world, according to the American Institute of Cancer Research, is due to the fact that majority of the U.S. population is obese and overweight, we tend to consume alcohol in excess, we are not paying enough attention to the foods we eat, and we do not engage in as much physical activities as we should.

Age—it is undeniable that your risk of developing certain types of cancer increases as you are getting older; these include breast cancer, colon cancer and prostate cancer just to name a few. Even though you cannot reverse the number of years you have lived, you can make some wise choices to lower your risk of developing cancer. It is never too late to pursue a healthy life.

Family history—only a small number of cancers are hereditary or are due to an inherited condition. If a certain cancer is common in your family, it is possible that mutations are being passed from one generation to the next. You might be a candidate for genetic testing to see whether you have inherited the mutations that might increase your risk of certain cancer. Keep in mind that having an inherited genetic mutation does not necessarily mean you will get the cancer.

Your health conditions—some chronic health conditions may increase your risk of developing certain cancers, these include but not limited to ulcerative colitis, certain esophagitis and polyps of the colon.

Your environment—certain harmful chemicals in the environment around you can increase your risk of cancer, for example, you might inhale second-hand smoke if you go where people are smoking or if you live with someone who smokes. Even if you are a non-smoker. Chemicals in your home or workplace, such as asbestos and benzene, are also associated with increased risk of cancer. Excessive exposure to sunlight can increase the risk of developing certain skin cancer.

Chronic inflammation—inflammation is a normal physiological response that helps injured tissue to heal. The process starts when chemicals are released by the damaged tissues. In response, white blood cells make substances that cause the cells to divide and grow to rebuild tissue in order to repair the injury. Normally, once the wound is healed, the inflammatory process ends.

In chronic inflammation, the process may begin even when there is no injury, and worse yet, it does not end. Chronic inflammation may be caused by infections that do not go away, an abnormal immune reaction to normal tissue or conditions such as obesity. Other situations that can cause chronic inflammation include changes in our intestinal flora that facilitate the growth of pathogenic or bad bacteria, yeast and fungus which keep our immune system in a state of alarm.

Stress can lead to chronic inflammation, though indirectly. Stress, whether physiological or psychological, can trigger the release of cortisol which can mobilize sugar and suppress the immune system, causing chronic inflammation. This is a double whammy situation because the high cortisol state can lead to insulin resistance, raising the risk for diabetes.

Over time, chronic inflammation can cause DNA changes and thus lead to cancer via mutations. For example, people with chronic inflammatory bowel diseases, such as ulcerative colitis and Crohn's disease, have an increased risk of colon cancer. Inflammation also plays a major role in many other diseases familiar to us. Just to name a few, arthritis, heart disease, asthma, chronic obstructive pulmonary disease (COPD), gum disease, gastrointestinal disease and skin disease like psoriasis. According to a 2015 study published in the Journal of American Medical Association, inflammation in the brain may be linked to depression and dementia.

Diet of bad foods—it is very true that you are what you eat! There are certain foods out there that can increase your risk of getting cancer. The most common ones are the processed foods which include bacon, salami, sausages and hot dogs. Scientists from ten different countries, after extensive research, concluded that eating processed meats—smoked, salted, fermented or preserved—increases the chances of developing bowel cancer. In fact, the World Health Organization, WHO, in 2015 stated that processed meats are as bad as smoking regarding the content of carcinogen. They placed hot dogs, sausages and other processed meats in the same category of cancer risk as asbestos, alcohol, arsenic and tobacco.

Meats cooked on a barbecue grill may create carcinogenic substances in the process of burning and grilling. So, go easy on the barbecue.

How about GMO? It stands for Genetically Modified Organisms, plants or animals, whose DNA has been altered in order to be resistant to pesticides and insecticides. While the Food and Drug Administration in our country and the biotech companies insist that GMOs are safe, many food safety advocates claim that these products have not had sufficient and satisfactory testing to determine their effects on humans. In fact, there is no direct data suggesting harm from eating GMOs. Some studies have shown that the use of pesticides even at low doses can increase the risk of certain cancers, such as leukemia, lymphoma, brain tumors, breast and prostate cancers. However, research into the link between GMOs and cancer remains inconclusive and controversial. But why accepting any risk at all when you can choose organic products, which by law exclude GMOs.

Hormone production in our body change as we get older. The endocrine system is made up of organs and tissues that produce hormones. Hormones are natural chemicals produced in one location, and released into the blood stream, then used by other target organs and systems.

Levels of most hormones decrease with aging, but some hormones remain at levels typical of those in young adults, and some may even increase. However, the endocrine function generally declines with age because hormone receptors become less sensitive. Some might consider hormone replacement therapy, but in some cases, such as estrogen replacement is potentially harmful in older women. Some evidence suggests that replacing certain hormones such as growth hormone in the elderly can improve functional outcomes, for example, muscle strength and mass, bone mineral density, but little evidence exists regarding effects on mortality, meaning they do not necessarily increase life expectancy.

Levels of melatonin, a hormone produced by the pineal gland, also declines with age. It is converted from serotonin via the enzyme, methyltransferase inside the pineal gland. The decline may play a role in the loss of circadian rhythm with aging. Melatonin is known to be a free-radical scavenger, and therefore an antioxidant with many health benefits including enhancement of the immune system.

As we get older, the levels of testosterone decline. Adults with diagnosed testosterone deficiency may benefit from testosterone replacement therapy. However, the effects of testosterone replacement therapy on coronary artery disease are not well understood, and it remains controversial.

Radiation-induced cancer is a real thing. In fact, up to 10 percent of invasive cancers are related to radiation exposure, including both ionizing and non-ionizing radiations. Most of the non-invasive cancers are non-melanoma skin cancers caused by non-ionizing ultraviolet radiation. Non-ionizing radiation can also come from mobile phones, electric power transmission, and other similar sources. In fact, these sources of non-ionizing radiation have been described as a possible carcinogen by the World Health Organization, even though the risk remain unproven.

EXPOSURE TO IONIZING RADIATION IS KNOWN TO INCREASE THE INCIDENCE OF CANCER, PARTICULARLY LEUKEMIA.

Obesity—this is a serious condition, a lot more than most people think, and is the cause of many illnesses including cancer. Many researches including data from the National Cancer Institute have shown that people who are obese may have an increased risk of several types of cancer, including cancers of the breast(especially in post-menopausal women), endometrium (the lining of the uterus), colon, rectum, esophagus, kidneys, pancreas and gall bladder.

Currently, a whopping 34 percent, or about 78 million Americans are obese, according to the Journal of American Medical Association. The statistics for children are not encouraging either, with 17 percent of those between 2 and 19 years old reported to be obese. If we can cut down the rate of obesity, we should see an improvement of cancer rate.

Sunlight—getting too much sun is dangerous, and skin cancer is a very real risk for anyone who spends extended periods of time without covering up or wearing appropriate sunscreen. Apart from this, spending some time in the sun with the proper precautionary measures is healthier than you think.

Women who spent the most time in the sun outlived those who avoided its rays, according to a recent study following 30,000 Swedish women for 20 years, taking smoking, exercise and obesity into consideration. The possible explanation is the vitamin D boost participants received resulting in improved cardiovascular health.

Alcohol—when consumed in moderation as recommended, it can have health benefits. The Federal Government's Dietary Guidelines for define moderate drinking as up to one drink per day for women and up to two drinks per day for men. Unfortunately, many people drink excessively and habitually, and for a few of them, it has become a dangerous, destructive addiction. This can increase your risk of cancer of the mouth, throat, esophagus, larynx, liver and breasts. Simply put, the more you drink, the higher your risk of cancer.

Tobacco—smoking causes majority of the lung cancer, which is the leading cause of cancer deaths in the U.S. for both men and women. Ironically, lung cancer is the most preventable form of cancer in the world. Besides lung cancer, tobacco-use also increases the risk for cancers of the mouth, lips, nose and sinuses, larynx, esophagus, stomach, kidneys, bladder, uterus, ovaries, cervix, colon and rectum.

In the U.S., cigarette smoking is responsible for nearly one in five deaths; this equals about 480,000 early deaths a year, according to the U.S. Surgeon General 2014 report.

By the way, cigars contain many of the same carcinogens found in cigarettes. Cigarette smoking causes huge economic losses, estimated about 300 billion dollars each year between 2009 and 2012 in the U.S., at least half of this money went for direct medical care of adults. (Sources : U.S. Surgeon General 2014 report).

According to Cancer Facts and Figures 2014, each year about 3,400 non-smoking adults die of cancer as a result of second-hand smoke.

Many people have the misconception that social smoking is safe as long as they don't smoke on a regular basis. They do not realize how damaging even light smoking is for their health, increasing their risk for cancer, heart disease, lung disease and many other medical conditions. According to a recent study from Sax Institute in Australia, even light, social smokers can double their risk of early death.

There are things you can do to avoid cancers or decrease your risk of developing cancers:

- Cutting down on sugar and junk (processed)foods. They cause fat buildup in your liver, which can cause liver damage and increase the risk of liver cancer. It has been predicted that non-alcoholic fatty liver disease will be the leading cause of liver cancer in the coming decades.
- Keeping your stress in check. Your immune system needs to be in optimal condition to seek out and destroy cancer cells. There will always be legitimate reasons to be worrisome or angry, but if your anxiety will not help the situation, then accept, adapt, and resolve things the best way you can.
- Adopting a Mediterranean diet supplemented by olive oil. Due to the anti-inflammatory property, this diet can help prevent cancer, according to many studies, including randomized trials published in the Journal of American Medical Association.
- Getting regular checkup. Be proactive because many cancers are curable or have a better outcome when discovered early. You can also do regular examination on yourself at home, especially self-breast examination for women.
- Getting vaccinated. There are vaccines available specifically to prevent some cancers. For examples, vaccines for HPV (Human Papilloma virus), hepatitis B and hepatitis C.
- Maintaining a healthy weight. Overweight and obesity have been linked with many types of cancers. So, do regular exercise, get enough sleep, eat your foods mindfully and choose foods low in carcinogens, and balance family and work. A report released on 05/14/2016 by the American Institute for Cancer Research and the World Cancer Research Fund warned that

alcohol, processed meats and obesity increase stomach cancer risk. The studies involved 17.5 million adults with those three factors of alcohol, processed meats and obesity and found 77,000 of whom were diagnosed with stomach cancers.

The researchers suggested that if everyone avoided the three risk factors they studied, Americans could prevent 4,000 new stomach cancer cases each year. Stomach cancer, also known as gastric cancer, is the fifth most common cancer and the third most fatal.

- Going beyond sunscreen. Sunscreen is the first defense, but it is not the only way to protect yourself from harmful ultraviolet rays. Wear a broad-rim hat and sunglasses with UV protection when you are outdoors. You must remember that prolonged exposure to the sun can hurt your health in the long run. Over the years, it can put you at risk for wrinkles, age spots, scaly patches called actinic keratosis, and skin cancers.

- Enjoying the nature. Gardening or walking in the wood is a good way to connect with nature to maintain a calm lifestyle and strengthen the immune system, not to mention about all those cancer-fighting antioxidants found in fresh fruits and vegetables.

- Be physically active on a regular basis. People who are physically active and doing exercise regularly live longer and have lower risks for heart disease, stroke, type-2 diabetes, depression and some cancers. Obesity and sedentary lifestyle have been linked to cancer-causing deaths, including two of the most common ones in the U.S., breast and colon cancers.

- Keeping your brain active. This will increase the level of connectivity between neurons in the brain and keep your brain healthy and reduce the risk of cancer.

- 80 percent rule. Keep your diet at least 80% plant-based with fruits and vegetables. It will lower the risk of some types of cancer and other chronic diseases, according to the Center for Disease Control and Prevention.
- Doing things that bring you joy. Living a happy life is just as important as eating well and exercising for a healthy life. Try to find things that make you happy, whether it is in your work or during personal time. It will further reduce your risk of getting cancer.

With the topic of inflammation receiving more and more medical attention and public interest due to its important role in many diseases, it is only natural that more and more people are looking into the so-called anti-inflammatory diet. Since inflammation and the immune system are closely intertwined, an anti-inflammatory diet should be a healthy, balanced diet with a focus on certain foods that have strong anti-inflammatory properties which can boost your immune system. However, if you have certain medical conditions in which inflammation may have a questionable role, you should inform and work with your physician while adopting a balanced, ant-inflammatory diet. Please be reminded that an anti-inflammatory diet, just like other positive lifestyle changes such as regular exercise, takes some time to work, and your patience and fortitude is necessary.

The following is a list of foods that have good ant-inflammatory properties:

- Tart cherries—in 2012, researchers from Oregon Health and Science University suggested that they have the highest anti-inflammatory content of any food.

- Berries—in general, all fruits can help fight inflammation because they are low in fat and calories, and high in antioxidants. The powerful chemical, anthocyanine, plays an important role in cell-repair. Studies show that women who eat more strawberries have lower levels of CPR, an inflammation bio-marker in the blood. Lab studies show blueberries may prevent cancer by slowing down growth of cells and reducing inflammation.

- Olive oil—researchers at the University of Pennsylvania have found that the chemical compound, oleocanthal, which gives olive oil its taste, in extra-virgin olive oil inhibits inflammatory enzymes in the same way that ibuprofen does. So, use some olive oil on your veggies and salads, or dunk your whole grain bread into it to reap its health benefits including reduction of your joint pain.

- Oranges—excellent source of vitamin C, potassium, fiber, calcium and folate. Vitamin C is very important for our immune system, strong connective tissues and healthy blood vessels. Eating oranges should be part of an anti-inflammatory diet.

- Grapes—they contain resveratrol which inhibits inflammatory enzymes in much the same way as aspirin.

- Papaya and pineapples—their enzymes, papain and bromelain respectively, in these tropical fruits, have been shown as effective as non-steroidal anti-inflammatory drugs, like ibuprofen and naproxen, for pain and inflammation.

- Dark chocolate—it contains chemicals that help fight inflammation. Its flavonoids act as antioxidants, protecting cells from harmful free radicals. Cocao contains polyphenol, an antioxidant with anti-inflammatory properties.

- Dark leafy greens—these include the common kale, spinach and broccoli. They contain vitamin E which may play a role in protecting the body from pro-inflammatory molecules called cytokines. They are also rich in phytochemicals, called glucosinolates, which are powerful antioxidants. Broccoli is my personal favorite of all the dark leafy vegetables; it is easy to prepare, just put them in boiling water for a few minutes before eating. Do not toss out the liquid part which contains a lot of nutrients. I drink it like a healthy beverage.

  Broccoli contains glutathione, an antioxidant that may guard against arthritis. Other fruits and vegetables high in glutathione include cabbage, cauliflower, asparagus, potatoes, tomatoes, avocados, grapefruits, peaches, oranges and watermelons.

- Nuts—such as almonds and walnuts, are full of omega-3 fatty acids, which have strong anti-inflammatory effects.

- Soy protein—researchers at Oklahoma State University found that people with osteoarthritis, who ate 40 grams of soy protein per day for three months had less pain and moved more easily than those who did not. Studies suggested that, isoflavones, compounds found in soy products may help lower CRP and inflammation levels. Soy protein can be found in soy beans, tofu and soy milk.

- Fatty fish—such as salmon, anchovies and mackerel are good sources of omega-3 fatty acids which have powerful anti-inflammatory properties. A University of Pittsburgh study found that people with back and neck pain who took omega-3 fatty acids in supplement form for three months had less pain overall. So, eat fatty fish at least twice a week and consider taking a daily omega-3 fatty acid supplement. I personally take 1000mg of fish oil in capsule form daily.

- Green and black tea—they are rich in antioxidants called flavonoids. Many studies have shown that these flavonoids can protect against cell damage and fight inflammation, reducing the risk of heart disease and cancer.

- Mangoes—this tropical fruit, not only nutrient-packed, but also a powerful inflammation fighter. One study in 2013 found that compounds in mangoes called polyphenols might inhibit the inflammatory response in both cancerous and non-cancerous breast cells. In addition to its anti-inflammatory benefits, they are a good source of over 20 vitamins and minerals including vitamins A, C, B6, folate and potassium.

- Garlic and onion—these pungent vegetables are powerful fighters against inflammation with similar effects to NSAID painkillers in our body like ibuprofen.

- Ginger and turmeric—these spices are common in Asian and Indian cooking. Many studies have proven their anti-inflammatory properties. Their antioxidants are boosters for the immune system.

- Beets—this red vegetable has powerful antioxidants which have been shown to reduce inflammation, as well as protect against cancer and heart disease., thanks to their contents of fiber, vitamin C and plant pigments called betalains.

- Tomatoes—they are rich in lycopene, which has strong anti-inflammatory properties. In a recent study from the Illinois Institute of Technology, IIT, subjects ate one meal containing tomatoes and one meal that did not have tomatoes. They were tested for a marker of inflammation after both meals; their inflammation levels were found to be significantly reduced after the tomato meals.

- Black peppers—they contain a powerful compound, called piperine with strong anti-inflammatory properties. No wonder black peppers have been used for centuries in Eastern medicine to treat multiple health conditions and maladies including pain. Recent animal studies have found that piperine may have the ability, not only to decrease inflammation, but also the ability to interfere with the formation of new fat cells, a reaction known as adidogenesis, resulting in a decrease in body fat, waist size and cholesterol; levels.
- Green and red peppers—these colorful vegetables should be part of a healthy diet. These hot peppers like chili and cayenne are rich in capsacin, a chemical that is used in topical cream to reduce pain and inflammation.
- Dry beans—such as navy beans, kidney beans and black beans, have many minerals, B-complex vitamins, protein and fiber. Their polyphenols work as antioxidants with excellent anti-inflammatory properties in addition to their many other health benefits.
- Sweet potatoes—including purple potatoes, are rich in vitamins and minerals. Like most orange-colored vegetables, they are high in vitamin A and carotene, which are powerful antioxidants. Along with their vitamin C and fiber, they are wonderful anti-inflammatory foods. In a study from Washington State University, the researchers found that men had reduced markers of inflammation after eating purple potatoes daily for six weeks.
- Low-fat dairy (yogurt with probiotics)—the probiotic can reduce inflammation. In addition to their anti-inflammatory properties, it is important to get their calcium and vitamin D for healthy bones and possible reduction of cancer risk. One

caveat: people with a diagnosis of rheumatoid arthritis are advised to consult their specialists about this.

- Avocados—rich in heart-healthy mono-unsaturated fatty acids. They are also good sources of many nutrients and polyphenols and avocados should be part of your anti-inflammatory diet.

As pointed out earlier in this chapter, inflammation and your immune system are intertwined, affecting each other. A healthy immune system is, not only necessary to fight inflammation in your body, but also important in reducing cancer risk. It is all the more crucial when you have a diagnosis of cancer because a strong, healthy immune system gives you a better chance to be a cancer survivor. In fact, there are many cancer patients enjoying the remission of their cancers following an anti-inflammatory, immune-boosting diet while undergoing medical treatments. Nutritional supports have become more and more important in many cancer treatment facilities in order to improve patients chance of survival.

Let us look at some of the foods that can boost your immune system and may help prevent cancer or, at the least, to reduce your cancer risk. If you already have cancer, it does not hurt to include these foods in your diet while you are receiving medical care from your physicians. More and more evidence are showing that the foods we eat weigh heavily in the war against cancers. The easiest and least-expensive way to reduce your cancer risk is simply by eating a healthy diet, according the experts at the National Institute of Cancer, at least 80% plant-based with fruits and vegetables.

- Grapefruits—they are high in vitamin C, which has been linked to a reduced risk of cancers of the stomach, colon, esophagus, bladder, breast and cervix. These research results are specific to vitamin C-rich foods rather than supplements.

- Leafy green vegetables—they are a good source of vitamin E. A 2012 study published in the Journal of National Cancer Institute found that vitamin E may protect against liver cancer. They also contain a phytochemical called indole-3 carbinol, which has been found to deactivate an estrogen metabolite that promotes tumor growth. Cancer protective properties of cruciferous vegetables like broccoli, cauliflowers and cabbages have been well-known. They all contain phyto-nutrients called glucosinolates, which may help inhibit the metabolism of some carcinogens and stimulate the body to produce detoxification enzymes. Their glutathione, an antioxidant, is a definite booster for your immune system.

- Carrots—like sweet potatoes, are rich in carotenoids, fat-soluble compounds that are associated with a reduction of several cancers. Their beta-carotene is converted into vitamin A in your body, mopping up the damaging free radicals to improve the immune system and the aging process.

- Sweet potatoes—they have many health benefits like their purple counterparts with their powerful, protective antioxidants. Regular consumption may help reducing the risk of breast cancer as much as 50 percent, according to some studies.

- Oysters—high in zinc content, which appears to have some virus-fighting powers. That is probably because zinc helps create and activate white blood cells in the immune response. It also assists your immune system with tasks such as wound healing.

- Button mushrooms—rich in selenium, B vitamins such as riboflavin and niacin. They play a role in a healthy immune system.
- Yellow potatoes—they are fattening when consumed in processed forms high in unhealthy saturated fat and salt, like French fries. A healthy form of potatoes is baked or boiled, its skins are rich in chlorogenic acid, a phytochemical that has been shown to have anti-cancer properties.
- Turmeric—a yellow-colored spice found in curry powder; curcumin is the ingredient of turmeric and has both the anti-inflammatory and antioxidant properties. In animal studies, curcumin has been shown to prevent cancer of the breast, colon, stomach, liver and lungs.
- D-fortified dairy products like low-fat milk and yogurt— they can protect against colon and breast cancers. Researches postulated that vitamin D may help block the development of blood vessels that feed the growing tumors.
- Peanuts—they are rich in vitamin E, which has been linked to a reduction of stomach, colon, lung and liver cancers. Almond is also a good source of vitamin E.
- Green tea—drinking at least three cups a day seem to have beneficial influence for breast cancer, according to a study in 2009. Green tea contains compounds called catechins that may help stop the growth of cancer cells. In Japan, where tea is the preferred beverage, green tea consumption has been linked to reduced risk of stomach cancer among women. In China, green tea drinkers were found to have a lower risk of developing rectal and pancreatic cancers, compared with non-tea drinkers, according to some pharmaceutical studies. So, start a habit

of drinking green tea instead of soda and you may enjoy its cancer-protecting influence among many other benefits.

- Soy including tofu—according to a report from the American Institute of Cancer Research, tofu may reduce the likelihood of breast cancer recurrence.

- Blueberries and pomegranates—they contain ellagic acid which may interfere with the metabolic pathways that feed certain cancers. Of all the fruits and vegetables studied, blueberries seem to be the most promising in reducing cancer risk. An antioxidant called pterostilbene, found in high quantities in blueberries, has cancer-fighting properties, according to some research studies. Anyway, all the berries including blackberries, cranberries, raspberries and strawberries contain powerful tumor-blocking compounds like phenolic acids, glycosides and anthocyanins that can slow the reproduction of cancer cells and stop free radicals from damaging cells.

- Seeds—including pumpkin seeds, flaxseeds and sunflower seeds, they all contain lignans which hinder estrogen production, thus limiting the spread of breast cancer. Based on many studies, dietary lignans can reduce risk of breast cancer and improve survival rate of breast cancer. Clinical evidence showed that women with breast cancer who ate the most lignans appeared to live longer.

Researchers from the University of Toronto conducted a randomized double-blind placebo-controlled clinical trial of flaxseeds, the world's most concentrated source of lignans, in breast cancer patients. They found that flaxseeds appear to have the potential to reduce human breast cancer growth in just a matter of weeks. Ground flaxseeds should be recommended to all breast cancer patients. As for women with high breast cancer risk, University of Kansas researches gave these women a teaspoon of ground flaxseeds a day for one year, and found a drop in pre-cancerous changes in the breasts.

Unfortunately, most women do not consume flaxseeds. Research showed that flaxseeds boost the activity of Tamoxifen to inhibit the inflammatory interleukin-1, which may help tumors grow and invade. Tamoxifen may reduce breast risk, but at the cost of severe side effects such as blood clots. Lignans are not a magic bullet to prevent breast cancer, but as a part of a healthy diet and lifestyle, they may help to reduce the risk of breast cancer in the general population.

- Legumes including green peas—a study published in the International Journal of Cancer showed that daily consumption of these lowers the risk of stomach cancer.
- Peppers—we already know their strong anti-inflammatory properties with their high contents of vitamin C and antioxidants. They also contain bioflavonoids, plant pigments that may help fighting cancer.

Some people may be skeptical and are not ready to accept the link between healthy foods and their protective properties to lower cancer risk and improve cancer survival. They probably want to see conclusive scientific findings which essentially are not possible with these epidemiological associations. Anyway, we are talking about a balanced, healthy diet with mindful eating, avoidance and reduction of unhealthy foods, and positive lifestyle changes. All of these can only benefit you, whether you have cancer or not. You should not let academic arguments prevent you from the pursuit of good health and a meaningful life journey.

There are things you can do and pay attention to for a better immune system:

- Try to kick back and relax whenever and wherever you can because stress can notoriously weaken your immune system,
- Get a pet, preferably a dog, for good companionship and exercise. This will lead you to better health.
- Find the time and mood to enjoy regular sex. Studies found that those who had sex in a relationship more often were in better health with longer life than others.
- Build a strong social network. Studies showed that loneliness weakened immune system. To improve your social circle, try volunteering, taking a class, or joining a group that interests you. And be sure to nurture the bonds you already have.
- Be optimistic. Positive thinking can boost your immune system. To increase your optimism, take time to savor the things you enjoy, look for the silver lining in tough, difficult situations, and try not to dwell on negative thoughts.
- Find something to laugh about. There is some evidence that laughter may help boost your immune system, and there is some truth to the famous saying: laughter is the best medicine.
- Eat your antioxidants. Remember the 80 percent rule for fruits and vegetables. To get a wide range, go for lots of colorful items.
- Keep your body moving. It is undeniable that exercise strengthens your immune system and decrease the risk of osteoporosis. You can do anything you like, as long as you are moving, such as walking, golfing, dancing, swimming, gardening, doing yoga, just to name a few.
- Avoid sleep deprivation. A good night's sleep makes your immune system stronger to fight off illness.

- Limit your alcohol because alcohol in excess weakens your immune system in addition to many other health problems it can cause.
- Do not smoke and avoid second-hand smoke. Kick the habit if you are smoker. There is nothing good about smoking, which increase your cancer risk of lung cancer and pulmonary diseases. It is very damaging to your immune system.
- Washing your hands. Use soap and clean with running water. Make sure that you wash them for at least 20 seconds in order to flush the germs down the drain.

CHAPTER THREE

Aging and the Mind

Our mind is a very ' precious thing ', but it can also be a very feeble ' thing '. Among the major public health concerns in the U.S., dementia is one of the top six, the others include heart disease, HIV/AIDS, smoking, obesity and cancer. Of the top 50 causes of death in America, according to data from HealthGrove, dementia and Alzheimer's Disease are among the top ten.

Dementia is a broad term for a group of symptoms including trouble with learning and memory, a chronic loss of cognition. Nowadays, we are hearing a lot about Alzheimer's Disease; Alzheimer's is one form of dementia, the most common type, accounting for at least 70 percent of all cases. Age is the number one risk factor; its actual cause is still not fully known or understood. Less than 5 percent of the cases are familial or hereditary. No vitamin, supplement, food or drug has been shown to cure this disease. Research suggests that your best bet is a diet rich in fruits, vegetables, fish and nuts to help protect your brain. There is no silver bullet!

Alzheimer's Disease can start many years before the symptom of memory loss. It is a debilitating neurological condition in which the dearest-loved ones can turn into strangers. The American Academy of Neurology estimate that the number of Americans affected by Alzheimer's Disease will triple over the next 40 years, adding up to about 14 million people in demand of an effective treatment that keeps them safe and helps maintain quality of life. Alzheimer's is not a normal part of aging, even though people who live to 85 or older may have up to 50% chance to have the disease. It is more common in women than men.

The two most common types of dementia affecting older Americans are Alzheimer's Disease and vascular dementia with Alzheimer's accounting for about 70% of the cases. Vascular dementia is caused by a series of micro-strokes that people are not even aware of most of the time. It has been well-established that hardening of the arteries, or atherosclerosis, is a risk factor for these strokes. Vascular dementia can be delayed and sometimes even prevented by diets that help lower blood pressure, decrease cholesterol and prevent or manage diabetes.

The signs and symptoms of Alzheimer's Disease are numerous and can be very subtle, developed over time. Some of them may not be readily apparent to family members or caregivers. It is not unusual for someone with the disease to become physically or verbally aggressive. Verbal outbursts, including cursing, arguing, name calling, shouting, and threatening are common; some patients will even get physical, hitting and pushing caregivers, for example.

The signs and symptoms of Alzheimer's Disease (AD) can get worse as the day goes on, called ' sun downing '. They can continue through the night, often resulting in sleep disorder.

At times, people with the disease can act like a child and become completely dependent upon a certain individual and constantly follow them around as shadowing.

You will notice a person with AD sometimes will make silly, irresponsible or even inappropriate decisions, a marked departure from his or her past behavior. For example, he or she is dressed inappropriately for the weather.

One of the earliest changes in judgment for people with AD is the handling of money. They might give money to unworthy strangers like telemarketers, or withhold money they should pay such as utility bills. They will have difficulty keeping track of the regular monthly bills.

We forget or misplace things sometimes. But people with AD might put the car keys in the freezer and the remote control in the drawer of the dresser. Although we are inclined to associate forgetfulness with the natural aging process, people with AD do not just occasionally forget where they left the car keys; they leave them in unusual places and are later unable to find them.

They can get confused with time or place such as forgetting where they live or where you live, getting lost easily and losing track of dates, seasons, and the passage of time. Many have a tendency to walk and wander aimlessly, and become lost many a times. In some cases, he or she might leave the house in the middle of the night to find a toilet for a physical need because they do not realize that they are home.

People with AD or dementia have trouble completing routine daily tasks that he or she has done them many time before. For instance, a former good cook in the kitchen may have a problem making his or her favorite dish, or even remembering how to boil water. In reality, they can literally forget to eat and drink, showing decreased appetite and interest in food.

Repetitive speech or action is a hallmark of dementia and AD.

Recognition does come and go for a while. As the disease progresses, your loved ones affected by AD may not always recognize you or other family members and friends. This can be very sad and heart-breaking! In the very late stages of the disease, patients may not even remember or recognize their parents.

People with dementia and AD will show difficulty with fine motor skills such as the ability to button or unbutton clothes or use utensils like forks and knives. They may forget the need to bathe or brush their teeth, leading to poor personal hygiene and grooming.

Unfortunately, the disease may progress to delusions and paranoia, both visual and auditory, making it harder and harder for caregivers.

Researchers have identified several types of brain abnormalities in people with AD, notably plaques made of clumps of beta-amyloid protein and tangles of a protein called tau. Both of these deposits correlate with the death of brain cells, leading to progressive memory loss, decreasing social skills and eventually, death. Alzheimer's memory loss goes beyond the usual " I forgot where I put my keys ". Memory loss is not consistent and people with AD may forget the dog's name one day and remember it the next day.

We start losing brain cells in the 20s; it is a normal part of getting older. There are things that can aggravate the age-related memory loss, such as smoking marijuana, high blood sugar, obesity and stress.

You can have memory problems weeks after smoking marijuana; it dulls your thinking, problem solving and physical coordination. Thus, it can cause learning difficulty.

According to a study published in the journal Neurology, people with high blood sugar, even those who do not have diabetes, may have an increased risk for developing cognitive impairment. Hippocampus is the part of the brain associated with memory and learning. Imaging studies confirmed that rising blood sugar was associated with decreased activity in the dentate gyrus section of hippocampus. Because blood sugar levels tend to rise with age, monitoring and taking steps to lower blood sugar as we grow older may be an important strategy for preventing age-related cognitive decline for everyone, not just people with diabetes.

The obesity epidemic is not only bad for our waistlines, but it can have a significant effect on our minds as well. Obesity is associated with difficulty in recalling past events, a poor episodic memory. It is also linked to a higher risk of dementia such as AD. The reasons for this are not clear, but it is known that obesity negatively affects cardiovascular health, which plays a vital role in brain health.

Studies have shown that the risk of developing Alzheimer's disease increased three times among individuals with the most saturated fat in their diet, and the risk increased five times for those who consumed a lot of trans fat.

The constant drumbeat of daily stresses can undoubtedly distract you and affect your ability to focus and recall. These stresses coupled with anxiety can lead to memory impairment.

In a survey of over 300 people participating in the Dallas Lifespan Brain Study, researchers found that among adults over 50, having a busy schedule was associated with better brain processing, improved memory, sharper reasoning and better vocabulary (ages from 50 to 89). Of course, being very busy could hurt cognition sometimes due to stress from maintaining a tight schedule. However, the data suggest that the benefits of busyness outweigh the downside. In other words, your brain will age better if you stay busy.

You can slow your age-related memory loss by staying active, such as exercise, dancing, reading, doing crossword puzzles and staying socially involved. More education such as learning something new is beneficial. Studies have shown that more mental stimulation through activities can lead to better memories. In other words, people who live busy lives have better memories.

Exercise is a good way to sharpen mental acuity. It can not only keep the brain focused on physical flexibility, motion sand coordination, but also can strengthen our cognitive capacities, including learning, memory, judgment, insight, mental clarity and focus. Exercise works like a medicine to increase the availability of neuro-transmitters like serotonin and dopamine in the brain which make us feel good and can prevent and treat mental illness.

Physical activity including walking can increase the release of brain-derived neurotrophic factor (BDNF), a protective protein in the brain, found to improve learning and memory according to many studies, in addition to its many other health benefits. BDNF, neuronal growth factor, plays a crucial role in neuroplasticity and cognitive function. Walking at a good pace has been shown to bolster the growth of new neurons; patients with Alzheimer's disease tend to have decreased BDNF levels compared to healthy, normal people.

Doing something new, or changing your routine can help your recall function. According to studies done by neuro-scientists at the National Institute of Health, when you are in a novel situation, your brain assumes that information is going to be important and hold on to it. So, taking a different route to work sometimes can help your recall function and boost your memory.

Studies published in the Journal of Alzheimer's Disease discovered that doing yoga or meditating at least once a week can help brain function and also prevent cognitive decline.

Studies have shown that laughing can improve short-term memory, especially for older adults, because laughing results in being less stressed, which can improve memory function.

You should consider writing notes instead of using the laptop, computer or cell phone sometimes. Studies have shown that taking hand-written notes helps you remember material better because it also forces you to pay more attention to the information at hand.

Getting sufficient sleep at night is crucial for good health and good brain function. Even a short nap during the day, about 20 to 30 minutes, if possible, can refresh and improve your brain function. Many studies have demonstrated that chronic sleep deprivation is associated with an increased risk of dementia and early death from any cause.

Normal aging does lead to gradual changes in many skills associated with thinking and memories. For example, you might find it harder to focus your attention and absorb information quickly. The slowdown in processing can lead to a jamming of information entering your short-term memory, reducing the amount of information that can be acquired and encoded into long-term memory. Some mental sharpness may be reduced with aging, such as forgetting the name of the person we just met or forgetting where you just put your keys or where you parked your care at a busy, crowded parking lot. However, if you struggle to follow familiar directions or difficulty balancing your check book at home as a person who manages household income and expenses, this is far more serious than ' senior moments!"

You can try some strategies as described below which can help enhance your focus and the ability to attend to the information presented to you and improve your memory as a result.

- If you find that you tend to become distracted easily during conversation, try talking with people in quiet environments without distractions.
- When someone is talking to you, look at the person and listen carefully. If you missed something that was said, ask the person to repeat it or to speak more slowly.
- You might want to paraphrase what is said to make sure that you understand it correctly and reinforce the information.
- You can improve your ability to focus on a task and screen out distractions if you do thing one at a time. Try to avoid

interruptions if possible. For example, if someone asks you something while you are in the middle of reading or working, ask if the person can wait until you are finished.

Other strategies to protect your memory include adequate sleep, learning new things, regular exercise and using your senses (visual and auditory). As a reminder, memory decline is NOT inevitable.

A large meta-analysis suggests that at least a dozen factors can help and mitigate dementia according to researchers at the Pacific Neuroscience Institute at Providence Saint John's Health Center in Santa Monica, California. The research, published in 2020 in The Lancet, identified 12 "potentially modifiable" risk factors; together, they account for about 40% of worldwide dementia cases. The 12 risk factors are:

- Less education
- Hypertension
- Hearing impairment
- Smoking
- Obesity
- Depression
- Physical inactivity
- Diabetes
- Low or lack of social contact
- Excessive alcohol consumption
- Traumatic brain injury
- Chronic exposure to air pollution

Researchers have identified a number of foods that could help prevent Alzheimer's Disease, or help lower your risk for the disease. To improve executive function, speed of perception, overall cognition and fact-based memory, total vegetable intake seems most important. For autobiographical memory and visual-spatial skills, however, total fruit intake is the key, according to NutritionFacts.org.

Let us look at some of the ' brain foods '; the following list is helpful but not meant to be complete. Nevertheless, earing well is good for your mental as well as your physical health. The brain needs nutrients just like your heart, lungs and muscles.

- Berries—these include blackberries, blueberries, strawberries and raspberries. They contain high concentration of antioxidants which have been proven to boost brain power and fight off free radicals. They can improve memory loss. A 2012 Harvard study found that women who ate at least one cup of strawberries and blueberries a week experienced a slower mental decline at least by 2 and a half years compared to women who did not consume them.

   A long running Nurses' Health Study followed more than 16,000 women age 70 and older found that those who ate more blueberries showed slower rates of mental decline. Brain scan in functional MRI imaging can show a difference in brain function as people eat blueberries. Researchers suggested that it is the polyphenol phytonutrients, special antioxidant plant pigment, that actually cross the blood brain barrier.

- Pumpkin seeds—they contain high content of zinc which has been shown to enhance memory and thinking skills.

- Broccoli—it is a great source of potassium, which is known to enhance cognitive function and improve brain power. Its glucosinolate can slow the breakdown of acetylcholine, which is necessary for the Central Nervous System (CNS) to function properly and keep your memories sharp.

- Nuts—a study published in the American Journal of Epidemiology suggests that proper levels of vitamin E in the body might help to prevent cognitive decline, particularly in the elderly. Nuts are a good source of vitamin E along with leafy green vegetables, asparagus, olives, eggs, brown rice and whole grains.
- Coffee—it has a few good surprises recently. Recent studies have shown that caffeine and coffee can be used as therapeutics for Alzheimer's Disease. The caffeine and antioxidants in the coffee may help ward off age-related memory loss. Research from the University of Innsbruck in Austria found that giving people two cups of coffee a day improved memory skills and neuron signaling to the brain compared to those who did not receive it.
- Eggs—a cheap source of many important nutrients including amino acids, vitamin A, calcium, phosphorus, potassium, iron and choline. Choline in the egg yolks is an essential brain nutrient that help cell signaling, promoting brain development and improving motor function and memory.
- Avocados—they are a good source of monounsaturated fatty acids (MUFA), omega-3 and omega-6 fatty acids which increase blood flow to the brain and aid in the absorption of antioxidants. MUFAs have been shown to be protective of nerve cells in the brain called astrocytes. Avocados are also full of vitamin E which protects the brain from free radical damage and vitamin K, which protects the brain from the risk of stroke.
- Spinach—full of folic acid and beneficial enzymes which can strengthen synapses, boost neuro-transmission, and slow down the effects of aging and dementia.

- Whole grains—they have a low glycemic index, meaning they release sugar slowly into the blood stream, keeping you mentally alert throughout the day with a steady supply of energy.
- Tomatoes—their powerful antioxidant, lycopene, helps protect against free radical damage to the brain cells which occur in the development of dementia such as Alzheimer's Disease.
- Kale—leafy green vegetables have been strongly associated with lower levels of cognitive decline. They are packed with folate and vitamin B6, the two vitamins which are protective of your brain health. Kale also contains many different flavonoids and vitamin K with anti-inflammatory and antioxidant properties.
- Maple syrup—a recent study published in 2015 found the sap from a maple tree has more than 100 healthy, anti-inflammatory properties that can stop the brain cells from tangling up and clumping together—a phenomenon that increase the risk of Alzheimer's Disease.
- Beets—these purple root vegetables contain lots of nitrates which increase blood flow to the brain. Decreased oxygenated blood is associated with dementia and poor cognition. Nitrates from beets widen the blood vessels and feed the brain in the frontal lobe. Researchers at the Translational Sciences Center found that giving older adults a daily dose of beet juice helped to increase blood flow to the area of the brain associated with dementia.
- Fatty fish—salmon, halibut, tuna, mackerel and sardines are anti-inflammatory with their omega-3 fatty acids, helping to lower the risk of heart disease, improve memory and brain performance, and fight depression, according to many studies including the one from the University of Maryland Medical Center. Essential fatty acids can't be produced by the body, and

you need to include them in your diet. In fact, studies confirm that frequent fish eaters experience slower rates of cognitive decline as they age. These oily fish are also packed with EPA and DHA which can decrease the risk of AD.

There are three types of omega-3 fatty acids: the types found in fish called EPA and DHA, seem to have the strongest health benefits. Another form known as ALA is found in vegetables, flax seeds and nuts like walnuts.

- Olive oil—in 2015, a team of researchers from Rush University Medical Center designed a diet plan to reduce the risk of developing Alzheimer's Disease by as much as 53 percent, called the MIND diet. Virgin olive oil is at the heart of the diet, thanks to the polyphenols floating within its viscous liquid. Studies have shown that these potent antioxidants can improve learning and memory in mice, and potentially can reverse the damage in the brain.

- Black currants—they are full of vitamin C, which is known to improve mental agility and protect against age-related brain degeneration including dementia and AD.

- Flax seeds—they are loaded with omega-3 fatty acids, fiber, protein and lignans. Studies have shown that flax seeds can reduce inflammation and promote healthy brain cells.

- Walnuts—including almonds and others, they contain plenty of unsaturated fatty acids, fiber, zinc, iron, calcium and vitamin E. They help improve heart and cognitive functions, sharpening your memory.

- Green tea—with its catechins, sterols, carotenoids and vitamins, it definitely can alleviate mental fatigue and boost your brain function.

- Dark chocolate—it contains many antioxidants, particularly the flavonols, which have been shown to improve circulation, stimulate the brain and slow cognitive decline.
- Capers—these unassuming buds from plants are full of quercetin, which stimulates memory by improving blood flow to the brain.
- Curry—animal studies have shown that curry's active ingredient, curcumin can actually clear away the Alzheimer-causing proteins in the brain called amyloid plaques.
- Sage—used in the 16th century to boost memory and cognitive function. This herb contains an enzyme called acetylcholinesterase that sparks neurotransmitters in the brain.
- Celery—it is one of the richest source of luterlin, a plant compound that may help lower the rate of memory loss, according to some studies. Celery also has anti-inflammatory properties, good for the heart and brain.
- Bone broth—the animal bones contain glycine which has been shown to help improve both sleep and memory, according to some studies.
- Chewing gum—a 2013 study published in the British Journal of Psychology found that it improved short-term memory, probably due to increased oxygen flow to the parts of the brain that make us pay attention.
- Rosemary—this delicious herb has been shown to improve memory and cognitive function with its scent alone. It also acts as an antioxidant, removing free radicals from the body including the brain.

The MIND diet—introduced in 2015 by researchers at Rush University Medical Center was created specifically to reduce dementia risk in older adults. MIND diet is a combination of DASH and Mediterranean diet; it includes ten brain-healthy food groups: leafy green vegetables, nuts, beans, whole grains, fish, poultry, olive oil, wine and berries, especially blueberries.

Researchers from Columbia University reported that eating a Mediterranean diet was linked to lower risk of Alzheimer's Disease; it is also associated with the subsequent course of the disease and outcomes. They found that the more the participants adhered to the diet, the longer they lived. Within five years, only 20% of those with high adherence to this healthy diet died, with twice as many deaths in the intermediate adherence group. In the low adherence group, within five years, more than half were dead, and by ten years, 90% were gone. By the end of the study, the only people still alive were those with higher adherence to the Mediterranean diet.

Our bodies are not designed to be able to absorb, digest and metabolize large amounts of single vitamins. They are designed to extract vitamins in the correct amounts from the food we eat. The foundation of the issue is to eat a well-balanced diet instead of focusing on single vitamins. If your loved one is not getting enough nutrition through the diet, your physicians may recommend taking certain supplements.

Almost 90% of older adults with dementia are not diagnosed. According to researchers from University of Michigan, North Dakota State University, and Ohio University, after studying more than six million Americans aged 65 and older, they found that 91.4% of these older adults with cognitive impairments consistent with dementia had not received a formal, medical diagnosis. In other words, 9 in 10 older adults with dementia do not know they have it.

Furthermore, the studies also showed that some demographics were more likely to not receive a diagnosis. According to the findings, the largest undiagnosed group despite symptoms consistent with dementia were black older adults. It is truly surprising that cognitive assessments and dementia screening are not routine during the annual check-up of older adults. Nobody can deny the importance of having some baseline cognition-related information available to healthcare providers of patients over 65 during medical encounter.

As a summary for this chapter, your brain changes as you age, but the central mission of your brain never changes. Its job is to help you make sense of the world and oversee your daily operations and life. As we experience the world, practice habits and learn new information, our brain change, grow new connections and repair broken ones. We all lose our keys and forget names sometimes, and these occur throughout our lives. It is important to know that there are other reasons lapses in memory occur like certain medications, lack of sleep, certain illness, and excessive alcohol.

Brain health refers to the ability to remember, learn, plan, concentrate and maintain a clear, active mind. By taking steps to help keep your brain and body healthy now, you can enhance your life and even help reduce some risks to your brain as you age.

Engage your brain now. Use it or lose it! The brain is like a muscle; when it is in use, it is a good, healthy feeling.

I would like to finish this chapter with some discussion about " brain fog ". What is brain fog? Medically, it is a constellation of symptoms reported by patients. The definition of brain fog is actually and ironically kind of unclear. Despite the ambiguity associated with its definition, it is still recognized by the medical professionals as a symptom worthy of attention and treatment.

In general, brain fog is a feeling of being somewhat disconnected or spaced out, mentally confused and lacking clarity, focus and concentration. You may have difficulty thinking clearly and quickly, impaired short-term memory, reduced attention span and forgetfulness. The day-to-day functional abilities may be compromised and limited, resulting in some problems at work or at school; other issues include problems driving, managing money and medications.

According to recent studies, up to a third of people who had COVID-19 developed ' brain fog ' that lasted six months after their diagnosis. The potential causes of brain fog are many, and the jury is still out there. If you are suffering from any of the symptoms that result in your feeling not quite right, you should see a doctor. There are many reasons why brain fog happens, and the best treatment plan is one that you and your healthcare provider arrive at based on the most likely cause of your symptoms

CHAPTER FOUR

Aging and Sex

More and more researches are showing that intimacy and sex are beneficial to your health and general well-being. Regular time behind closed doors can make you look and feel younger, reduce your stress, boost your immunity, enhance your sleep and protect you against prostate cancer and improve your cardiovascular health. The landmark Masters and Johnson Study in 1986 links increased quality of life with the fulfillment of sexual desire.

A 25-year study from Duke University found that the more sex you have, the longer you will live. Furthermore, a recent study published in the Journal of Age and Aging found that having an active sex life over the age of 50 can boost brain health and eventually protect you from dementia. Researchers speculate that sex increases levels of feel-good hormones like dopamine and oxytocin in the brain.

Is your sex life aging well? According to surveys, about 50% of people over the age of 50 think so. A study in 2014 by the American Sexual Health Association showed that most people felt happy and healthy when their sex life was healthy. Though sexual activity does decline as you get older, many seniors stay sexually active. According to Kinsey Institute, 25% of men over 50 say they have sexual intercourse three to five times a month, and 10% say they have intercourse two to three times a week. The frequency of sexual intercourse for women are somewhat less in comparison.

As a matter of fact, the sex lives of older people often benefit from more experience and sexual confidence, and from relationships that have matured to a higher level of trust and intimacy. With aging, that may mean adapting sexual activity to accommodate physical, health and other changes. There are different ways to have sex and be intimate; the expression of your sexuality can include many types of touch or stimulation. Sadly, many older adults have difficulty adapting to changes and become asexual because they are set in their ways.

Safe sex and sexually transmitted diseases, STD, apply to both young and old; seniors are just susceptible to STDs as anybody else. In fact, the number of seniors with HIV is on the rise, so are cases of STDs like chlamydia, herpes and hepatitis B among seniors.

Usually, it takes longer for older people to get aroused. That does not mean you are out of the game. The couple need to be more creative and patient, with an open mind and attitude.

It is undeniable that seniors face certain challenges to a satisfying sex life. Some health issues may get in the way, like vision and hearing—which often carry sexual cues—can fade. Chronic illnesses can cause problems for your sex life, especially among older people. Diabetes, prostate surgery after cancer and other major surgeries, severe arthritis, memory loss or your partner's dementia can all negatively affect the sex life of seniors.

Chronic pain can interfere with intimacy between older people, but it can often be treated. Unfortunately, some pain medications can interfere with sexual function; you need to talk with your prescribing doctor if you experience such side effects.

For women, menopause with decreased levels of hormones, estrogen, testosterone and progesterone, can cause vaginal dryness and thinning, making intercourse uncomfortable and sometimes painful. This will adversely affect women's sex drive (libido) with less and less desire for sexual intercourse. Lubricants and lubricated condoms can often help in such situation. Furthermore, with reduced sexual sensation, women experience fewer and weaker orgasms. However, studies have shown that as many as half of post-menopausal women continue to enjoy good quality of life despite these physical and physiological changes.

Incontinence among older people is often embarrassing and inconvenient. One strategy is to go to the bathroom before you have sex. Your body has changed over the years. As you age, it is not unusual to become more insecure about how you look and appear to your partner. You might try to have sex in the dark to make you feel less self-conscious about your body.

The levels of the male hormone, testosterone, go down gradually with age. In some men, their testosterone levels can get so low causing less interest in sex, erection dysfunction, low energy and depression.

Erectile Dysfunction, ED, is one of the most common problems for men. It happens where there is not enough blood flow for your penis to get hard. Or when the veins that normally drain blood from it can't close up to keep the blood in and keep it erect. ED can happen to any men, but if you have certain health issues such as heart disease, a stroke, or diabetes, you are more likely to have it.

There are different causes of erectile dysfunction (ED) :

It is estimated that at least 40 percent of men with ED have hypertension and other cardiac diseases. The drugs that are used and prescribed to treat ED, unfortunately and ironically, can exacerbate hypertension and related heart problems such as angina pectoris.

The same can be applied to diabetes, a disease with associated abnormal arterial and nerve damages. It is not surprising to find 30 to 50 percent of men with diabetes report some form of sexual difficulty such as erectile dysfunction and decreased libido.

Obesity, with all of its complications and co-morbidities, is clearly a major cause of erectile dysfunction. Many obese people are living with metabolic syndrome, which is a cluster of medical conditions including obesity with abdominal or truncal fats, unhealthy cholesterol and triglyceride levels, high blood pressure and insulin resistance. They are likely to suffer from ED and poor libido.

An enlarged prostate, medically called benign prostatic hypertrophy (BPH) is a common cause of ED. It occurs in 60% of men over the age of 60 and 80% of men over the age of 80. This medical condition can be treated with medications prescribed by physicians. Others may require surgical intervention due to problematic symptomatology and potential cancer risk. Oftentimes, prostatic surgeries can worsen ED as one of the unpleasant complications affecting human sexuality. Of course, with the advance in medical/surgical technologies, the complications have been greatly minimized.

Many neurological diseases that affect the Central Nervous System (CNS) can cause ED. These include Parkinson's disease, multiple sclerosis and stroke, to name a few. These neurological conditions interfere with the functions of nerves as a result, adversely affecting sexual performance. Spinal cord tumors, spina bifida and polio have also been linked to Erectile Dysfunction.

Hormonal disorders can be a contributing factor to ED, most commonly, low levels of testosterone. This medical condition can be found in up to 10% of men. The low level of testosterone can be related to abnormal pituitary gland, abnormal thyroid and adrenal glands. It is important for you to check with your primary care physician and specialists to rule out any organic pathology for your low levels of testosterone.

Many physical injuries can directly cause erectile dysfunction due to damages to the nerves and blood vessels. One example is pelvic fractures from an accident like a fall, or motor vehicular accident. Certain activities such as riding a bicycle or horse-back riding can be a risk factor for ED, because of the potential damages to the nerves and blood vessels (veins and Arteries) in the pelvic floor.

Some surgeries can cause ED as one of the un-intended and unexpected complications. These surgeries include colo-rectal surgeries to treat cancers, and orthopedic surgeries in or near the pelvis. During surgeries, the nerves and blood vessels vital for sexual function may be affected or damaged. This post-operative erectile dysfunction may be short-term.

Certain prescribed medications can increase the risk of ED; these include some prescriptions for hypertension, heart problems and high cholesterol. Some psychotropic drugs for depression and bi-polar disorder are known to cause ED as one of the adverse reactions. Some medications used in chemotherapy and hormonal therapy can also be a culprit.

Many medical experts believe that much of the ED problems are caused by psychological conditions like anxiety and depression. This, as you can see, is becoming a vicious cycle: anxiety and/or depression can lead to ED, and ED can cause anxiety and/or depression. So, the inability to perform sexually is closely intertwined with some psychological overlay in some cases. When this is the underlying issue, you should seek professional help and guidance.

Vitamin D deficiency may play a role in erectile dysfunction, according to some recent studies, though not directly. Vitamin D is crucial for healthy heart function. A poorly functioning heart can lead to impotence. Men with vitamin D deficiency were 32% more likely to suffer from ED than men with higher levels, according to research presented at the 2015 annual meeting of the American Heart Association. The researchers said those findings reflect the effect that vitamin D has on vascular function including blood vessels that carry blood to the genitalia. In the journal of Sexual Medicine, Italian researchers linked vitamin D deficiency to dysfunctional blood vessels and lower levels of nitric oxide.

Recent studies from Harvard University found that low levels of vitamin B12 can be associated with erectile dysfunction.

About 40 percent of the people with obstructive sleep apnea (OSA) or other chronic pulmonary diseases suffer from ED, probably due to low oxygen levels in the blood.

Certain lifestyle habits can impact your sex life adversely, resulting in ED and decreased libido. These include alcohol which acts as a depressant in your body and nicotine which is a vaso-constrictor decreasing blood flow to the sex organs. Smoking is known to be associated with low sex drive, according to some studies.

Since we know that sex is desirable and healthy, and crucial for human relationship and a longer life span, let us look at some of the foods that can help with your libido and sexual performance in your journey of aging.

- Garlic—ancient Egyptians used garlic to boost their stamina. Researchers have confirmed that garlic helps stop the formation of fat deposits, called nanoplaques, inside arterial walls, including those leading to your penis. It also increases your circulation via an enzyme called nitric oxide synthetase, promoting more blood flow down there.
- Coffee—studies have shown that drinking two to three cups a day can improve erectile dysfunction. This holds true even for overweight, obese and hypertensive men, but not for those with diabetes, a condition that often causes ED. Researchers suggest that coffee, a stimulant, triggers a series of reactions in the body including increased heart rate, and ultimately improving blood flow to the penis. " Moderate coffee drinking keeps things going strong ".
- Nuts—including walnuts, peanuts and pistachios. They are a great source of heart-healthy omega-3 fatty acids. A good functioning heart promotes good sex. They also contain the amino acid, L-arginine, which is one of the building blocks of

nitric oxide for vasodilatation. Their high fiber content helps to bring down cholesterol levels keeping the blood vessels healthy.

- Blueberries—this super-fruit makes things harder in a good way. They are a great source of flavonoids, which are associated with a reduced risk of erectile dysfunction. According to a joint study from the University of East Anglia and Harvard University, of the six main types of flavonoids, three in particular— anthocyanins (in blueberries), flavones and flavanones (both found in citrus fruits) offer the greatest benefits in preventing ED.

- Oysters—loaded with zinc, which is a mineral that increases levels of testosterone and growth hormone. They also contain D-Aspartic acid, an amino acid shown to boost testosterone levels and improve sperm quality. With its high content of vitamin B12, oysters enjoy a reputation for being great for love and fertility.

- Clams—they are rich in vitamin B12 and L-arginine, an amino acid that converts to nitric oxide to open up arteries to the penis.

- Mussels—they are rich in vitamin B12 and magnesium, natural enhancers of erection.

- Chocolate—it is a sensual food, from its taste to its aroma. Dark chocolate has been shown to cause a spike in serotonin and dopamine, which produce the feeling of pleasure. Its flavanols, phytochemicals, can increase blood flow and help your body make more of nitric oxide.

- Green tea—its catechins, not only help burn belly fat, they also boost desire by promoting blood flow to your nether regions. The antioxidants also help get rid of the damaging free radicals in the body.

- Peppers—they contain the feel-good compound, capasacin, promoting sexual arousal. They also rev up your metabolism, making you sweat and speeding up your heart rate, thus, increasing blood flow to all essential areas.
- Cherries—this superfruit is packed with many vitamins, potassium, folate, iron, magnesium and more, which promote general and sexual health. They are a good source of the plant chemicals called anthocyanins which clean your arteries of plaques, keeping them open for business.
- Pomegranate—studies published in International Journal of Impotence found that pomegranate juice, which is rich in antioxidants, improve blood flow and can help with ED.
- Oats—They are a good source of L-arginine which increases production of nitric oxide. Their high fiber content help lower cholesterol levels, decreasing the risk of atherosclerosis. Simply put, the better your cholesterol level, the better your erection will be.
- Watermelon—it is rich in lycopene which has Viagra properties, relaxing the blood vessels to improve circulation to the crucial areas. Its high content of L-citrulline, an amino acid that can improve the strength of erection. Once in the body, it converts to L-arginine, stimulating the production of nitric oxide.
- Ginseng—it is famous for its many beneficial effects on health. Many studies had shown that it has strong vasodilatation property, improving circulation to all vital organs of the body. Researchers at the University of Hawaii found that women who took ginseng regularly experienced significant improvement in their libido. Thus, ginseng can be a natural alternative to Viagra for both men and women.

- Honey—it contains boron, which has a libido-enhancing effect. One study showed boron put women's sex drive into overdrive and increased men's testosterone levels.
- Pesto—the pine nuts are a great source of zinc which can improve sex drive. They are also rich in magnesium, which can raise levels of testosterone and help keep sperm healthy and viable. Magnesium is also a relaxer for blood vessels and muscles.
- Figs—this plump fruit is packed with amino acids involved in the production of nitric oxide, which relaxes blood vessels and increases blood flow to the sex organs. It causes penile and clitoral erections, vaginal lubrication and other parts of the sexual cascade, from desire to orgasm. So, add a couple of figs to your banana smoothie for a double dose of aphrodisiac. Biblically, figs were used by Adam and Eve in the Garden of Eden for procreation.
- Spinach—it is a good source of magnesium, which relaxes arteries and promotes blood flow to the genitalia. Optimal blood flow below the belt means more stimulation and stronger erection.
- Fatty fish—like salmon and herrings, have heart-healthy fat. They are also rich in vitamin B12 and magnesium which boost the production of testosterone. Along with their vitamin D, these fish can help you get and keep it up.
- Bananas—they are a good source of potassium, which counteracts the effects of sodium in salty foods, which can not only decrease blood flow to the genitalia, but also make it more difficult to reach orgasm. The enzyme, Bromelain, in bananas can trigger production of testosterone. Their vitamin B12, along with potassium, help increase energy levels for better sex.
- Arugula—this leafy vegetable contains many phytochemicals and antioxidants that can promote libido. Antioxidants can

remove oxidative damage to the vascular system caused by free radicals in the body—a process called natural rusting. This, in turn, provides a healthy environment for our organs and tissues.

- Artichokes—this vegetable enjoys legendary aphrodisiac reputation. It is packed with many vitamins and antioxidants which are important for proper body functions and good blood flow.
- Apple and apple cider—these rosy red fruits have a pretty timeline of history. Eve from the Garden of Eden could not resist taking a bite out of the forbidden fruit. Besides their anti-aging, cancer-fighting, immune system boosting properties, apples may have a romantic role in the bedroom.

There is no retirement age for desire, and sexual desire does not dissipate with age. Older people have sex for the same reasons anyone else does: pleasure, intimacy, fun, togetherness and excitement. Sexuality is at the core of who we are and has an impact on our lives in many ways. It does not stop once we reach the age of 60, 70, or 90, even 100 despite the myths and assumptions of society and certain cultures.

Unfortunately, the issues of sexuality with older adults often become a taboo topic. In the long-term care facilities, the expressions of sexuality are often labelled as problematic behaviors. The health care team rarely addresses those issues, even though there is a need to raise the awareness of the complex issues surrounding sexuality of older adults.

So, heat up some apple cider, add a spoonful of cinnamon (a proven aphrodisiac), and a few clover sticks (another sex stimulant), and enjoy the wonderful benefits of human sexuality!

CHAPTER FIVE

Aging : Looking Healthy and Youthful

Many people through the years, including kings and queens, and emperors and empresses in the past had tried to reverse the body clock of aging, looking for immortality. Our modern scientists and medical experts have been studying and attempting to turn the biological clock back without success, at least at this time. Others have been trying to stop the aging process of humans with very limited satisfactory results.

However, most of the researches have shown that we can maintain optimal functioning of different organs in our body for a long time with a balanced healthy diet which is 80% plant-based with fruits and vegetables, avoidance of known risk factors in the environment, a healthy lifestyle, appropriate exercise and physical activities, and beneficial mental stimulation.

As you know, you are unable to change the genes your parents already passed on to you that give you the unique look, anatomical features and stature. Some people, for the pursuit of perfection and vanity, did alter some parts of their body, thanks to the technological advances of modern medical science in the area of cosmetic-reconstructive surgeries.

Of course, this is strictly a personal choice and perception, except for certain medical situations where reconstructive surgical intervention is necessary as a therapeutic treatment.

In order to age well with healthy, happy and youthful appearance, we need to pay attention to several important areas : your hair and skin, maintaining a healthy body weight with well-balanced diet and physical activities, and a functioning, optimistic mind.

Let us start with your hair because aging changes in hair is definitely a clear and obvious sign of aging. Hair color is due to a pigment called melanin, produced by the hair follicles. Follicles are structures in the skin that makes and grow hair; when you get older, the follicles make less melanin, causing gray hair.

So, turning gray is one of the many changes your hair goes through as you age. Prolonged exposure to the sun can damage both your hair and skin with its ultraviolet rays, UVA and UVB. The rays destroy the outside cover of the hair strand, called cuticle and its protein, keratin. Signs of sun damage to your hair include dry and brittle strands, discoloration, broken or split ends, and thinning.

The only living part of your hair exists inside the hair follicle, and the hair you see is actually dead. Hair aging can be caused by microscopic, biochemical or hormonal changes that affect the follicles, or environmental factors that cause wear and tear on the hair itself. The onset of graying is determined by genetics. By age 60, 2/3 of men have significant hair loss. Women may experience baldness as they age, resulting in thinning hair and a visible scalp. It may be due to genetics, shifting levels of hormones, vitamin deficiency or certain health conditions. Other signs of aging hair include dryness due to shrinking oil glands in the skin, loss of hair volume leading to thinning of hair, and decreased rate of hair growth.

The sun's rays act very much like bleach biochemically on your hair; the bleach reacts with the melanin pigment in the hair and removes the color in an irreversible reaction.

The common hot flat irons and rollers, and chlorinated water in swimming pools can also make your hair vulnerable to the summer stresses of heat and sun. The damaged layer of cuticle allows sun and heat to penetrate the hair more easily, resulting in fragile hair strands.

There are a few steps you can take to protect your hair, especially during the summer:

- Go out early or late in the day, before 9am or after 3pm.
- Wash your hair two to three times a week, depending on your activity and weather conditions with a sulfate-free shampoo.
- Wear a hat or use an umbrella to cover yourself.
- Comb your hair when it is dry and not wet.
- Cut down your use of hot hand tools like flat iron and rollers.
- When blow-drying, keep the dryer at least 6 to 10 inches away from your head.
- If you swim in a chlorinated pool in public places, make sure you rinse thoroughly the pool water—which contains salt and chlorine—out of your hair with clear, warm water.
- You can use a hair conditioner, appropriate to your hair and type.

Healthy hair is an indicator of your overall physical wellbeing. It takes some time, months and years, to grow your hair to a long length; it is estimated that hair grows between ¼ and ½ inch per month. So, it can be a challenge to grow your hair and improve its quality due to the amount of time it takes to grow. What you eat and how you take care of yourself will be reflected in your hair. In other words, healthy-looking hair is a product of your lifestyle.

A well-balanced, healthy diet will do wonders for your hair, along with the non-diet measures. Staying hydrated and eating whole, nutritious foods can help your hair looking good and growing healthy.

The following is a list of some foods that are beneficial to your hair:

- Brazil nuts—they are a good source of selenium, which is a mineral important in almost every aspect of the human body including hair growth. Just two of them is enough to meet your daily recommended requirement. Selenium is also a powerful antioxidant which plays a critical role in DNA synthesis and helps protect your body from oxidative damage and infections
- Swiss chard—it is a great source of biotin, which is crucial for the growth of hair and nail. Please be patient with it because it takes months to see satisfactory results.
- Fatty fish—such as salmon, tuna, mackerel and sardines. They are high in omega-3 fatty acids, which are beneficial to the health of your scalp, among their other health benefits. They help balance the oils in your body, reducing flakiness and itching on your head. These essential oils will keep your scalp

and hair hydrated. The body needs them to grow hair and keep the hair shiny and full.

- Carrots—rich in vitamin A, which is important for proper hair growth. It can be best absorbed with a little healthy fat.
- Meats—including lean beef and lamb. Their zinc and protein content helps stimulate hair growth with thickness, while their iron content can fuel hair growth. They are a good source of vitamin B12, which can lead to significant hair loss if you do not have enough of it in your body. The iron in meat is a very important mineral for hair. Anemia is a major cause of hair loss.
- Eggs—the bad reputation of eggs seems to be fading because we are finding more and more health benefits with this common, inexpensive food. The high contents of protein in eggs along with biotin help hair growth, and you will have much to gain just eating one hard-boiled egg a day.
- Nuts—like walnuts, pistachios and almonds, their high vitamin E content has been shown to help hair grow faster. In fact, it is one of the viable treatment options for male pattern balding. You can massage the vitamin E oil from the supplement onto your scalp to improve circulation and stimulate hair growth.
- Citrus fruit—foods that are high in vitamin C, such as oranges and lemon can help reduce excess oil on the scalp and protect the structure of your hair. In particular, grapefruit juice can help strip your hair of buildup, and its vitamins A and C help boost hair growth.
- Dark leafy greens—like spinach and broccoli with lots of vitamin C, folate, vitamin A, minerals like iron, and antioxidants including beta-carotene can definitely provide the nutrients your hair need to grow in healthy manner.

- Chicken breast (without the skin)—including turkey. Eating sufficient protein every day is vital for the quality of your hair. Chicken has low fat and high protein, a very good and inexpensive option to keep your hair in healthy shape.
- Greek yogurt—it is packed with protein, the building blocks of hair. It also contains vitamin B5, pantothenic acid, which can help with blood flow to your scalp, thus may help against hair thinning and loss.
- Oysters—rich in zinc and vitamin B12, both of which are crucial for health of your hair. As already mentioned, low levels of zinc are associated with hair loss.
- Sweet potatoes—they are packed with antioxidants called beta-carotene, which the body converts into vitamin A to protect against dry, dull hair.
- Cinnamon—it is known to increase blood flow, delivering more oxygen and nutrients to the hair follicles for optimal hair growth.

The skin is the largest organ of the body, and is also the first line defense for us from external factors. It plays a key role in protecting the body against pathogens and excessive water loss. Its other functions are insulation, temperature regulation, sensation and the production of vitamin D.

The skin located under the eyes and around the eyelids is the thinnest skin in the body, and is one of the first areas to show signs of aging such as wrinkles. Years of exposure to the sun causes elastin in the skin to break down, leading to sagging and stretching of the skin. Other common skin changes as you age include age spots, freckles, and discolored blotches.

We all need to take precaution to protect our skin from the sun; people who need to be especially careful in the sun are those who have:

- Pale skin
- Blond, red or light brown hair
- Have been treated for skin cancer
- A family member who has had skin cancer

How common is skin cancer? It is the most common cancer nowadays. About 5.4 million basal and squamous cell skin cancers are diagnosed each year. Melanoma is the most deadly type of skin cancer, accounting for over 75,000 cases of skin cancer annually. And the number of cases continue to rise in 2016, and is anticipated to exceed 76,000 cases.

Protection from the invisible ultraviolet (UV) radiation is important all year round, not just during the summer or at the beach. Please be reminded that UV radiation is everywhere: it can reach you on cloudy and hazy days, as well as bright and sunny days. UV rays also reflect off of surfaces like water, cement walls of buildings, sand and snow. Indoor tanning beds, booths or sunlamps all expose you to UV radiations.

In the continental U.S., the most dangerous time for UV exposure outdoors is between 10am and 4pm, taking all the time zones into consideration. The Center for Disease Control and Prevention recommends some easy ways to protect yourself from UV radiation:

- Stay in the shade, especially during mid-day hours
- Wear clothing that covers your arms and legs
- Wear a hat with a wide brim to shade your face, head, ears and neck

- Wear sunglasses that wrap around and blocks UVA and UVB rays
- Use sunscreen with sun protection factor (SPF) 15 or higher and for both UVA and UVB
- Avoid indoor tanning

Special note: UVB rays are much stronger during the summer and are mostly responsible for your burning. UVA rays are weaker, they can contribute to both skin aging (wrinkles and brown spots) and skin cancer. They can penetrate clouds and the windows of your office and car. You may want to consider using sunscreen every day, year round.

Moreover, you should check your skin regularly, so that you know what is normal for you and to notice any new changes or new growth. Your cosmetics should offer protection from the UV rays.

The need for sun safety has become clearer over the past two to three decades. Many studies have shown that excessive exposure to the sun can cause skin cancers. Harmful rays from the sun, sunlamps and tanning beds can also cause eye problems, weaken your immune system and give your skin spots, wrinkles and leathery skin.

Things that can damage your hair, most likely can also damage your skin. For example, chlorine, which is a chemical used in swimming pools and to treat drinking water, can strip the natural oils of skin, causing it to become dry and crack.

If you are dehydrated, you will have tight, dry and flaky skin.

Over-exfoliating can cause self-inflicted damages to your skin, even though removing dead skin cells on the surface is commendable. You must exercise discipline and not exfoliate more than 3 to 4 times a week to avoid the risk of inflammation.

The area surrounding your eyes is very fragile with very thin skin. Avoid over-rubbing your eyes to prevent broken blood vessels.

Stop using the straw can help prevent wrinkles around the mouth. Sipping through a straw can accentuate those facial muscles where fine lines may appear.

Using silk pillow case for sleep will decrease the friction on your facial skin, unlike pillow cases made of cotton and polyester.

Try to sleep on your back, because sleeping on your side can cause the cheek to be pressed against the pillows increasing the chance of wrinkle formation.

Avoid taking hot, long showers because the hot water will remove essential moisture and oils from the skin causing it red, dry and flaky. This can aggravate conditions like eczema and rosacea.

Washing your face before going to sleep is critical for your skin health because the makeup, oil, and other chemical impurities can block your pores and lead to breakouts. Furthermore, this will disrupt cell turnover, a reparative process of your skin during sleep.

Smoking causes early aging of skin and premature wrinkles. In fact, researchers have documented the aging effects of smoking on the skin and have even coined the phrase ' smoker's face '. The multiple toxic chemicals in tobacco smoke damage the skin in many ways, affecting its elasticity, texture, color and even its chemical make-up. These damages leave the skin more vulnerable to cancer such as squamous cell carcinoma as well as non-cancerous psoriasis. Smoking has been shown to worsen skin conditions like eczema. People exposed to second-hand smoke also face a greater risk of these skin problems.

According to a 2009 study published in the Journal of Dermatology, cigarette smoking accelerates the rate of skin aging by producing more of the destructive enzyme called matrix metalloproteinase (MMP), which breaks down collagen fibers. Less collagen, more wrinkles. Collagen has been named the scaffolding that supports the outer layer of skin.

While it is true that many cosmetics including lotion and cleaners offer a topical fix—a beauty bandaid. A glowing complexion of smooth, hydrated skin starts from within. Americans spend over 55 billion dollars a year on their appearances, according to a 2014 report on the cosmetics industry. People spend plenty of time and money on their hair and skin. But there are many ways you can achieve aesthetic benefits without a salon or a pill—naturally through the food you eat. Other protective measures for healthy skin include retinoic acid, avoidance of air pollutants, stress reduction, moisturizers and a healthy diet.

Many foods, which are easy to find with your mindful approach, can nourish your skin and get that healthy glow you are after, despite the fact that your lifestyle habits (smoking and tanning) and genetics can certainly influence and predispose your skin to pesky conditions.

Let us look at some of the foods for your skin:

- Tomatoes—their famous phytochemicals, lycopene, help boost collagen strength. It is collagen, a protein, that gives skin its taut, youthful structure. Lycopene can also help fight off the oxidative effects of ultraviolet rays by eliminating skin-aging free radicals.
- Carrots—they have plenty of beta-carotene and vitamin A which are important for the health of your skin. Vitamin A also plays a role in reducing development of skin-cancer cells.
- Sweet potatoes—beta-carotene, which your body converts to vitamin A, a nutrient that helps skin shed dead cells, and protect against dry, flaky hair. It also boosts production of sebum in the scalp. A diet rich in fruits and vegetables, especially carotenoid –rich ones like sweet potatoes will give your skin a healthy, golden glow. So, do not hesitate to include this colorful veggie in your diet.
- Dried apricots—they are available in stores all year round. Their vitamin A plays a crucial role in promoting the growth of healthy new skin cells.
- Chicken, preferably breast without the skin—this staple poultry contains zinc and selenium, the minerals, that boost collagen production and maintain hormonal balance.
- Eggs—the egg yolk contains many B vitamins including the ' beauty ' vitamin, biotin. Biotin is known to help hair grow and strengthen nails. It is also healthy for skin.
- Oysters—as already mentioned for growth of hair, they contain high levels of vitamin B12 and zinc. Our skin cells rely on zinc, an important trace mineral, to make the protein to

repair damaged tissue and regenerate new ones. Zinc also has antioxidant properties.

- Cucumber—very high water content, at least 90%. Hydration is an essential part of maintaining beautiful skin. This plant also contains silica, a nutrient that aids the body in producing hyaluronic acid, which helps skin cells maintain moisture.
- Dark chocolate—its flavanols are potent antioxidants, which can reduce roughness in the skin and provide sun protection from UV radiation. Chocolate is also a great source of pre- and probiotics to help heal your gut and decrease inflammation.
- Flaxseeds—these little things have plenty of health benefits. They are rich in omega-3 fatty acids, which can alleviate inflammatory skin issues and improve overall hydration of your skin cells.
- Oranges—universally known for their vitamin C content, which is not just good for your DNA with its antioxidant properties, it is also important to keep your skin healthy. They are also full of wrinkle-fighting collagen for your skin. Most mammals can make this vitamin in their body, unfortunately, humans lost this ability many, many years ago. You can opt for lime or lemon if you don't like oranges.
- Almonds—they are full of vitamin E, which help repair damaged cells and defend against sun damage. Vitamin E is a potent antioxidant which helps keep your body free of harmful free radicals. Vitamin E is known to boost your immune function with its anti-inflammatory property.
- Walnuts—consuming just 5 grams of monounsaturated fatty acid (MUFA) may be able to lower the risk of skin cancer or slow its development, according to a study by the American Society for Nutrition. So grab a bag of walnuts and enjoy them as snacks

everywhere including while driving in your car. They are also packed with alpha-linolenic acid (ALA), an omega-3 fatty acid which reduces loss of water and nutrients from your skin cells, and helps fight inflammation in the form of scaly skin.

- Whole wheat bread—it has low glycemic index. During a 10-week Korean study of subjects with mild to moderate acne, researchers found that those placed on a low-glycemic diet decreased the severity of their acne more so than subjects on a high-glycemic diet.

- Brazil nuts—a rich source of selenium, which can boost the production of collagen. Selenium also helps preserve elastin, a protein that keeps your skin smooth and tight. They are also full of vitamin E to keep your skin moisturized.

- Oats—they are high-fiber foods that feed your inflammation-fighting gut bacteria, minimizing spikes in blood sugar that can contribute to skin problems. Oats are a good source of silicon, a trace mineral that helps skin retain elasticity, slowing the signs of aging.

- Nalto—a Japanese dish of boiled and fermented soy-beans. An excellent source of vitamin K2—a vitamin which is important for cardiovascular and bone health as well as promoting skin elasticity to prevent wrinkles. You can also get K2 from grass-fed butter, meat and egg yolks.

- Turmeric—many studies have shown that it can protect against cancer and reduce pain. This Indian spice can also protect your skin. Its active antioxidant, curcumin, is one of the most effective anti-inflammatory and free-radical fighting options out there. Studies have shown that this powerful pigment, curcumin, can prevent shortening of the telomeres. The shorter the telomeres get, the more likely you are to experience cellular aging.

- Coconut water and oil—when you first crack it open, you can drink the natural water of the fruit—it is full of muscle-relaxing potassium and electrolytes to replenish and re-hydrate the skin. Its oil and flesh contain a potent anti-microbial, caprylic acid, which can help improve gut health by destroying bad bacteria.

- Green tea—it contains catechins, antioxidants with proven anti-inflammatory and anti-cancer properties. Drinking two cups of green tea a day helps prevent skin cancer according to some research. Be careful to not overdo it because too much caffeine can lead to dehydration, which may have adverse effects on your skin.

- Kale—this dark green cruciferous vegetable is loaded with the favorite nutrients for skin health, the anti-aging vitamins A, C, E, and K. Vitamin K, when applied topically, can minimize the visibility of bruises, scars, stretch marks, and the unsightly spider veins.

- Blueberries—like strawberries, raspberries and blackberries, are loaded with antioxidants, which are powerful fighters against your body's cell-damaging, skin-aging free radicals. The anthocyanins help boost the strength of collagen fiber. It strengthens, in particular, blueberries, the immune system and alleviate inflammation-induced skin conditions. Their vitamin C helps prevent the wrinkling effect of sun damage.

- Salmon—this popular fish, besides being a great source of heart-healthy omega-3 fatty acids, salmon also contains dimethyaminoethanol (DMAE). DMAE promotes healthy skin because it protects the integrity of cell membranes, thjus guarding against premature aging. DMAE also helps to prevent the production of arachidoric (AA),an inflammation precursor that leads wrinkle formation. In addition, salmon is also a good source of niacin, a B vitamin that keeps skin healthy, and selenium, an antioxidant that helps protect your skin from sun damage.

- Papaya—a tropical fruit containing many beneficial enzymes. One is chymopapain, a strong anti-inflammatory. Another enzyme, papain, can help remove blemishes and even treat acne when applied topically as the enzyme dissolves pore-clogging fats and cleanses the skin. Papaya is also rich in vitamin C, which is a collagen-strengthening vitamin; it is also one of the most potent antioxidants for protecting the skin from damage that can lead to wrinkles.

- Pineapple—it is rich in a mineral, called manganese, which is needed to activate prolidase, an enzyme necessary for the production of proline, an amino acid. Proline is an integral part of collagen, which helps your skin maintain strength and elasticity to ward off wrinkles and fine lines.

- Yellow peppers—their high content of vitamin C is essential to the formation and growth of skin and muscle tissue as well as to building collagen—the protein which provides strength and structure to your skin, bones, muscles and tendons. The British study in the American Journal of Clinical Nutrition found that volunteers who ate yellow peppers daily, even a couple of bites, for three years decreased the appearance of wrinkles by 11 percent.

- Spinach—in a study published in the International Journal of Cancer, people who consumed the most leafy greens had half as many skin tumors over the course of eleven years compared to those who ate the least of the veggies. Spinach is also rich in folate, an essential B vitamin for good health. Its high content of the vitamin A precursor, beta-carotene, helps fight off the free radicals and prevent skin damage. Spinach is really a nutritional super-star with its other health benefits.

- Avocado—it is rich in mono-unsaturated fatty acids (MUFA) which protects the skin against ultraviolet radiation, thus lowering the risk of premature aging. Its fats also help you absorb many of the fat-soluble vitamins that are beneficial for your skin.

- Water with slices of lemon or orange—this mixed drink is known as ' detox water '. The vitamin C in the citrus will help balance the levels of electrolytes and expel excess water weight while d-limonene acts as a powerful anti-inflammatory compound which aids the liver flush toxins from the body.

- Watermelon—it is packed with lycopene which acts as a natural sunblock. Its high water content also helps to your skin hydrated.

- Ginger : it is packed with strong anti-inflammatory properties which may help reduce puffy eyes, and your aches and pain.

I find it helpful to use the Healthy Hair and Skin Index to serve as a quick guide in rating the beneficial levels of 30 foods; in general, the higher the number, the better for your skin and hair.

Foods	Healthy hair/skin index	Main nutrient
Sweet potatoes	93	Vitamin A
Red bell pepper	92.3	Vitamin C
Kale	91.7	Vitamin A
Collard Greens	91.4	Vitamin A
Papaya	91.2	Vitamin C
Beets	91.0	Vitamin A
Butternut squash	90.6	Vitamin A

Spinach	90.2	Vitamin A
Rainbow trout	90.2	Vitamin D
Pacific oysters	89.6	Zinc
Swordfish	89.4	Vitamin D
Butter melon	89.3	Vitamin C
Pumpkin	89.2	Vitamin A
Sockeye Salmon	88.9	Vitamin D
Orange	88.6	Vitamin C
Carrots	88.2	Vitamin A
Strawberries	88.0	Vitamin C
Lima Beans	87.4	Vitamin C
Brussels sprouts	87.2	Vitamin C
Broccoli	86.3	Vitamin C
Red grapefruit	86.3	Vitamin C
Pea pods	85.8	Vitamin C
Lemon	84.7	Vitamin C
Sunflower seeds	84.5	Vitamin E
Green peas	83.3	Vitamin C
Almonds	82.1	Vitamin E
Cranberry juice	82.1	Vitamin C
Clams	81.7	Vitamin C
Zucchini	81.6	Vitamin A
Pacific halibut	81.6	Vitamin D

In order for you to age well with a healthy and youthful look, you must not be overweight or obese. A Gallup survey published in February of 2016 showed that the obesity rate among adults in the U.S. surged in 2015 to a new high of over 32 percent. When you add the 35 percent of Americans who are overweight to this, you have about 67 percent of the adults in the U.S. who need to maintain a healthy weight.

Overweight and obesity will cause many medical problems for you over time, including diabetes, heart disease, high blood pressure, hyperlipidemia, chronic aches and pain, sexual dysfunction and low self-esteem just to name a few. Obesity has certainly reached an epidemic proportion in the U.S. and deserves our serious attention. But it is not within the scope of this book to deal with the overweight and obese problems in details.

Nevertheless, the major reason for obesity and overweight to have become such a significant health problem in the U.S. is the foods many of us consume every day. To maintain a healthy weight, you need to cut down on sugar and salt. You also need to avoid packaged and processed foods including regular and diet sodas. You must follow a balanced diet which should be 80% plant-based, meaning 80 percent of your meals coming from vegetables and fruits.

Maintaining a healthy weight also requires positive lifestyle changes without unhealthy personal habits such as smoking, drug abuse and alcohol drinking in excess. You have to do exercise on a regular basis about 120 to 140 minutes a week if possible; there are many forms of exercise for different age groups and it is not hard to find physical activities that you will enjoy and can handle physically.

When you get older, sometimes it can be depressing because your children have grown and left home to live their own independent lives. You may feel lonely and isolated at times. That is why it is important for you to stay socially connected with friends and do things with them. Try to have a positive attitude and outlook because you will not look good and healthy if you are depressed and unhappy.

CHAPTER SIX

Aging and Longevity

The word " longevity " is sometimes used as a synonym for " life expectancy ". To be precise, the term " longevity " usually refers to especially long-lived members of a population, whereas " life expectancy " is defined statistically as the average number of years remaining at a given age.

Around the world, certain groups of people enjoy exceptionally long lives. The Pacific Islanders of Okinawa, Japan, have an average life expectancy of more than 81 years, compared to 78 in the U.S., and a world-wide average of just 67. Here in the U.S., members of the Seventh Day Adventists, who typically eat vegetarian diets, outlive their neighbors by 4 to 7 years on average.

Residents of the San Blas Islands off the coast of Panama very rarely suffer from hypertension and heart disease. Indeed, researchers show that their rate of cardiovascular disease is only 9 percent per 100,000 people, compared to 83 per 100,000 among the Panamanians on the mainland. More and more evidence suggest that diet is one of the important contributors to longevity and healthy aging.

Knight Templar's secret of longevity might lie in their unique diet, according to researchers. Their diets required eating lots of fruits, vegetables, dried legumes and fish rather than meat, and drinking moderate amount of wine with aloe pulp. Their diet enabled them to live mush longer compared to the people of the Middle Ages, whose life expectancy averaged 25 to 40 years.

Longevity has been a topic not only for the scientific community, but also for writers of travel, science fiction, and utopian novels. There are many difficulties in authenticating the longest human life span ever by modern verification standards, due to inaccurate or incomplete birth statistics. Fiction, legend, and folklore have proposed or claimed life spans in the past vastly longer than those verified by modern standards.

The world population continues to grow at an unprecedented rate. Today, about 9 percent of people worldwide are aged 65 and over. This percentage is projected to jump to at least 17% of the world's population by 2050, with the number of seniors totaling more than 1.6 billion.

Well, we know that humans around the world are living longer, and life expectancy in most countries has increased due to advances in healthcare, agricultural techniques and decreased infant mortality. But that does not necessarily mean that we are living healthier. The increase in our aging population presents some public health challenges that we need to prepare for. In the U.S., the 65 and over population is projected to nearly double the next three decades, from 48 million to about 90 million by 2050. The global life expectancy averages out to 71.4 years, according to the most recent statistics. That means that some parts of the world see much shorter life spans, while others enjoy greater longevity.

Let us look at the five ' blue zones ' of the world where centenarians are common:

Okinawa, Japan—a gregarious, closely-knit community with considerable social support through all of life's ups and downs, thus, reducing mental stressors and reinforcing shared healthy behaviors. It is not surprising to find many of the women living well past the age of 100.

Loma Linda, California, U.S.A.—this U.S.'s only blue zone is a haven for the Seventh-day Adventist Church, a Protestant denomination. Their emphasis and shared principle of community and adherence to the Sabbath—a day of rest, reflection and recharging—help resident-Adventists of Loma Linda live at least 10 years longer than their fellow Americans. It is noteworthy that many avoid meat and eat plenty of plants, whole grains and nuts.

Sardinia, Italy—a mainly plant-based diet, daily physical activity and familial closeness have given this Blue Zone the highest concentration of male centenarians in the world. Most of the men are sheep herders, who tend to walk at least five miles a day. It also does not hurt that the M26 marker, a genetic variant linked to extreme longevity, has been passed down through generations in this secluded community.

Nicoya, Cost Rica—the residents of this Blue Zone in Costa Rica tend to avoid processed foods, and traditionally the Costa Ricans get the majority of their calories from beans, squash and corn, plus tropical fruits. Their plant-based nutrient-dense diet with plenty of outdoors activities promote strong, well-nourished bodies; along with devoted, guiding life purposes, many Nicoyans stay mentally and spiritually fulfilled to age 90 and beyond.

Ikaria, Greece—a strong sense of self-respect and pride keeps Ikarians invested and involved in this island community. A strict adherence to the Mediterranean diet including lots of fruits, vegetables, beans, whole grains, red wine, etc. keeps the islanders of Ikaria healthy, both physically and mentally, with longevity.

The richest Americans live at least 10 years longer on average than the poorest, in general. According to studies by Princeton University, men with the top 1 percent income level lived 15 years longer than men with the lowest 1 percent in income, for women that gap was 10 years. Interestingly, while the income does decide your life expectancy to some extent, the locality in which you reside, your lifestyles and the foods you eat also decide how long you will live.

In a cohort study, the combination of a plant-based diet, normal BMI (body weight within normal range), consuming alcohol in moderation as recommended, and not smoking accounted for differences up to 15 years in life expectancy. Other additional lifestyle factors that promote longevity and improve aging included sleeping 7 to 8 hours per night and healthy snacking between meals. There are, however, many other possible factors potentially affecting longevity, such as the impact of high peer competition typically experienced in large cities, drug abuse and intense contact sports.

There are other simple things that can help you add years to your life:

- Brushing your teeth at least three times a day, including flossing; this helps decrease bacteria and inflammation.
- Simple walking for 20 to 30 minutes after dinner in your neighborhood can improve your life expectancy.

- Having a positive attitude with an optimistic approach will bring more happiness in your life, and happiness is strongly related to how long you will live.
- Making new friends and expanding your social network is good for your general well-being, promoting a long, healthy, and meaningful life-journey.

Women normally outlive men, and this was as true in pre-industrial times as today. Theories for this advantage include smaller bodies (and thus less stress on the heart), a stronger immune system (since testosterone acts as an immune-suppressant), and less tendency to engage in physically dangerous activities. In other words, men tend to take bigger risk. Furthermore, men die of heart disease more often than women and at a younger age statistically. Men commit suicide more often than women unfortunately, and I think this is due to the fact that men are less likely to be socially connected.

Another social factor in the difference of 5 to 6 years in the life expectancies of men and women is: men tend to avoid doctors and medical screenings. Do not forget that human genetics favor women. The Y chromosomes tend to develop mutations more often than the X chromosomes, and the lack of a second X-chromosome in men means that X-linked abnormalities among boys are not ' masked ' by a second normal version. It is not surprising that by age 85, at least 67% are women.

Let us look at the life expectancy chart listed by the World Health Organization in 2013, for the countries in the world, and for the sake of simplicity, I will show the top 25 countries, and surprisingly, the U.S. is ranked the 34th in that year with a life expectancy of 78.5, a combined figure of men and women, despite that fact that we are the wealthiest and most influential nation in the world.

Name of country	Overall rank	Life expectancy
Japan	1	84 years
Spain	2	83 years
Andorra	2	83 years
Singapore	2	83 years
Switzerland	2	83 years
Australia	2	83 years
Italy	2	83 years
San Marino	2	83 years
France	9	82 years
Monaco	9	82 years
Republic of Korea	9	82 years
Iceland	9	82 years
Israel	9	82 years
Canada	9	82 years
Cyprus	9	82 years
Luxembourg	9	82 years
New Zealand	9	82 years
Norway	9	82 years
Sweden	9	82 years
Austria	20	81 years
Greece	20	81 years
Finland	20	81 years
Portugal	20	81 years
Germany	20	81 years
Netherlands	20	81 years

In June, 2021, the list shows some minor changes in rankings, with Japan still has the longest life expectancy at 84.2 years, while Switzerland has the second spot at 83.3 years, Spain at 83.1 years and Australia 82.9 years for the top four positions.

It is undeniable that tobacco use, alcohol and drug abuse, insufficient consumption of fruits and vegetables, low level of physical activity along with sleep deprivation, will directly or indirectly, contribute to the global burden of aging, including here in the U.S. The fact that Japan and many other countries spend less than the U.S. on healthcare per capita, yet see their people living longer, is a clear indicator that the Land of the Free should do something differently.

A diet abundant in nutrients with fruits and vegetables is obviously important to longevity and healthy aging. Studies of centenarians the world over also suggest that social connections and finding meaning in life are both crucial to longevity. Getting older can come with a variety of health challenges because age is a real risk factor undeniably and unfortunately. But you can take action to maintain good health and reduce your risk of disease and disability now. It is never too late. The chances of discovering one major pill or potion to fight off all the effects of aging are very slim and probably unlikely, but you yourself can control many aspects of healthy aging.

Research has shown that you can turn back the biologic clock by making a few science-backed changes to your diet and daily habits. One key has to do with telomeres—bundles of DNA that cap the chromosomes. The longer your telomeres, the less likely you may be to develop conditions like cardiovascular diseases, obesity, diabetes dementia and many cancers.

Telomeres naturally shrink with age, but studies have shown that it is possible to curtail the process and even lengthen your telomeres by making diet and lifestyle changes, according to Harvard research. If you go organic, the lengthening of telomeres is even better, according to a major analysis published in the British Journal of Nutrition. Added sugar such as sugary beverages have been implicated in cell aging, leading to shorter telomeres, according to a study from the University of California, San Francisco. Scientifically speaking, you can slow down the aging process at the cellular level!

Another huge factor is inflammation : it is the common denominator in many diseases such as arthritis, type diabetes, cardiovascular diseases and Alzheimer's Disease. Aging is associated with increased inflammation, but as with telomere length, certain lifestyle habits can help prevent and even reverse the inflammation that lead to premature aging and decline, and development of disease.

Before we get to the foods that promote longevity, let us look at the non-diet things that may help you live a longer, meaningful and enjoyable life. As a reminder, your genes only have about a 10% influence on how long you will live. Experts say that the choices you make throughout your life are much more important.

- Feeling younger than your real age is good for longevity, according to a recent British study. The findings were so powerful and astounding that ' feeling older ' was linked to increased risk of dying by 41%. That is why marrying someone is linked to living longer, according to some studies.
- Maintaining a positive attitude is associated with longevity, according to a study of centenarians in 2012 in the journal

Aging. Researchers from the Albert Einstein College of Medicine at Yeshiva University found a correlation between optimism and longer life span. A positive attitude toward life can be the difference between checking out early and being the last one at the party. This positive trait can add up to 7.5 years to your lefe span, according to some studies.

- Taking an afternoon nap promotes longevity. Harvard researchers studied more than 23,000 people for six years and found that those who took a 30-minute siesta had a 37% lower chance of dying from heart disease than those who stayed awake all day.

- The practice yoga is relaxing with cumulative effects of lower blood pressure, less stress, a healthy weight, less anxiety and less breathing can lead to a longer life span. Or, getting a body-mind routine with Tai Chi, which can enhance and promote many health benefits and is recommended by the U.S. Department of Aging.

- Sleeping naked can slow the aging process, but not too many of us do that. It is estimated that only 12% of Americans have the healthy habit of sleeping naked. The reparative growth hormones are more effective at cooler temperature. Being cooler also decrease the levels of cortisol in our body.

- Be conscientious. In their book, The Longevity Project, authors Howard and Leslie Martin wrote that being conscientious was one of the best predictors of a long life. They postulated that people who are diligent and responsible may be more likely to adopt healthy behaviors, may be less prone to disease and may find more success in relationships and in the workplace.

- Quit smoking. This is really a no-brainer. We all know all the bad things about cigarette smoking; in the U.S. alone, there are 480,000 premature deaths related to smoking annually. Research published in the Journal The Lancet followed 1.3 million people between 1996 and 2001. The study showed that giving up cigarettes helped participants live 10 years longer than of they had continued smoking.

- Avoid prolonged sitting (no more than three hours). People who spent an average of six hours a day watching TV died nearly five years earlier than people who did not watch any TV at all, according to research from the University of Queensland, Australia.

- Cooking more at home, at least 4 to 5 times a week. This makes you live longer than those who eat out or order takeout most of the time, according to a study published in Public Health Nutrition in 2012.

- Move to a higher ground. A 2011 study from the University of Colorado School of Medicine found that 20 U.S. counties with the highest life expectancy had an average altitude of 5,967 feet above sea level, with a gain between 1.2 and 3.6 years.

- Physical activities including walking. According to a 2012 study in the Archives of Internal medicine, of 19,000 middle-aged adults, regular exercise and/or physical activities can decrease the risk of developing Alzheimer's, certain cancers, heart disease, and type-2 diabetes in their 70s and beyond. In other words, people who remain active throughout their life span live longer, according to studies by Johns Hopkins University School of Medicine. If you enjoy walking, you might want to consider doing some weight lifting which is more helpful for your bone health than walking, especially for the post-menopausal women or older women.

According to a 2011 JAMA Internal Medicine study, women ages 65 to 69 who break a hip are five times more likely to die within the next year compared to older men. Furthermore, the greatest risk of death occurred in the three months following the fracture.

- A new study over a 14-year period in Psychological Science found that people who feel they have a sense of purpose in life are less likely to die. So, go and make new friends, pick up a new hobby, or volunteer. A meta-analysis of adults over age 55 found that regular volunteers were 24 percent less likely than others to die over the course of the study. Feeling useful may help your brain make more oxytocin and progesterone which help decrease stress and inflammation.

- Connections. Stay socially engaged and connected is important for a long, meaningful life because social isolation often can lead to chronic illness and depression. Friendship is the key in Sardinia, Italy, a tiny Mediterranean island with a large centenarian population. A long list of friends may add years to your life. One study found that people with many chums lived 22% longer than those with only a few. Loneliness is actually bad for you; it can lead to memory loss, depression, anxiety and chronic illnesses. Your closest friends do not have to live close to you. Research shows that distance does not harm friendship strength or benefit. A phone call to a friend far away can make you feel connected and this connection can decrease loneliness and stress. Tel Aviv University researchers followed 820 adults for 20 years and found that those with the most social support lived the longest.

- Try to keep up your sex life. Many studies have shown that sex is important part of life and health. A healthy sex life can lengthen your life span.

- Keep your brain busy. Your brain likes something to puzzle over and figure out. It loves making new connections and learning. More and more research shows that a healthy brain into old age depends on constant intellectual stimulation. A busy brain is good for longevity. So, take some classes, learn new things and stay smart.

    A 2008 WebMD survey found that 89% of centenarians keel their minds active. And being creative can add more time to your life expectancy. Research published in Science journal in 2013 suggested that expanding your horizon could help expand your brain and might prevent life-shortening dementia.

- Take control of your medical care. Not understanding your medications and treatments can raise your risk of death. Studies have shown that patients who do not ask questions or do not understand their medical conditions are at an increased risk of complications and death. It is important for you to take time to research and understand your medical conditions because it can save your life!

- Getting yourself tested. You need to make a commitment to keep up with the preventative care and screening plan you have with your physician. When an illness or a medical condition is detected early, the rate of success and cure is the highest.

- Get a pet. Pets are not just great companions to beat loneliness, they can actually help you meet human pals, too. One study shows people who own dogs, cats or other pets are more likely to know the folks in their neighborhood. They also get interactions and advice from people they meet through their pets.

- Openness is a good trait. Willing to lend an ear to new and different ideas, feelings and concepts is linked with a long life.
- Take the stairs if you can. Researchers from the University of Geneva calculated that many people with a sedentary lifestyle simply taking the stairs was enough physical activity to burn body fat and lower blood pressure—enough to cut their risk of an early death by 15%.
- Meditation. Many studies have shown that it can help improve many types of conditions, including depression, anxiety, chronic pain, diabetes and hypertension, as well as improving concentration, memory and reasoning skills.
- Avoid sunburn. Sun exposure is crucial for your natural production of vitamin D, which is associated with a few health benefits such as stronger bones and a lower risk of some cancers. As with everything, moderation with sun safety in mind is the key.
- Slowing your resting heart rate is a key predictor of long life in otherwise healthy middle-aged and elderly men, according to Danish researchers, probably due to less stress on the heart.
- Get married. Married people tend to outlive their single friends. Even people who are divorced or widowed have lower death rates than those who have never tied the knot.
- Try to be forgiving. Chronic anger and bitterness is linked to diminished lung function, heart disease, stroke and other ailments. Forgiveness will decrease anxiety, lower your blood pressure and help you breathe more easily. All these will promote a longer life. So, don't go to bed angry!
- Use safety gears. Accidents are the fifth most common cause of death in the U.S. Seatbelts reduce the chances of death or serious injury in a car wreck by 50%. Many deaths from bicycle accidents are caused by trauma to the head; so always wear a helmet.

- Get spiritual. People who attend religious services tend to live longer than those who don't. The strong social network that develop among people who worship together may contribute to the overall health due to improved immune system, according to researchers. According to a review of research published in 2006 in the journal of American Board of Family Medicine, going to church weekly can add 1.8 to 3.1 years to your life expectancy. The review further found that if you join the choir, you will get the same health benefits as yoga due to the calming effects on the mind and body.
- Brush and floss your teeth. You have got more than cavities to worry about if you do not brush and floss as often as your dentist recommends. Poor oral hygiene has been associated with shortened life expectancy because maintaining a healthy oral environment, your mouth, can lower risks for heart disease, dementia and stroke.
- Washing your hands with appropriate soap or cleaners for at least 20 seconds is life-lengthening. According to a 2005 study by the World Health Organization, the simple act of hand-washing could save more lives worldwide than any vaccine or other medical intervention.
- According to a study published in the Journal of Rejuvenation Research, intermittent fasting may increase longevity-boosting genes. If you can manage intermittent fasting occasionally, I do not see any harm done, as long as you are not going to make up for what you miss overeating.
- Taking more vacation. According to the analyses of the famous Framingham Heart Study, they found that the more frequently men took vacations, the longer they lived.

- Remember the 80% rule of mindful eating. Stop when you are 80 percent full. Ben Franklin said: ' Lessen thy meal, lengthen thy life '.

Retirement is not resting and staying still. Don't retire from life when you are retired from your career. It should be the time for you to try to reach optimal health and work toward a long life of wellness and happiness. Be sure that you are ready to take care of your mind and body for the years to come.

There are many healthy foods out there if you just open up your mind and eyes, but I am going to list some of them and call them ' Longevity Foods'.

- Grapefruit. Among those 65 and older, one out of five falls causes a serious injury like fractures of bones, major or minor, according to the Centers for Disease Control and Prevention. Though you have heard that drinking milk can help keep your bones strong and healthy, so can grapefruit juice, say Texas A&M University researchers. Studies have shown that grapefruit juice can improve bone density and slow the rate of bone loss.
- Blueberries. They are packed with antioxidants that give them their purple or deep red color. They protect the cells from damage by changing the way neurons in the brain communicate and reduce the accumulation of protein clumps most frequently seen in Alzheimer's. In one study, adults supplemented with blueberry juice for just 12 weeks scored higher on memory tests than those receiving placebo. So, a diet high in blueberries can stave off memory loss by several years.

- Spinach. It is superbly green and leafy. It is a rich source of plant-based omega-3 fatty acids and folate, which help reduce the risk of heart disease. stroke, and osteoporosis. The folate also increase blood flow to the nether regions, helping to protect you against age-related sexual issues.
- Cruciferous vegetables. Broccoli, cabbage and cauliflower are loaded with vitamin C and other important nutrients; people who consume them regularly tend to live longer lives.
- Grapes. These little things are filled with anthocyanins, which help fight arthritis and boost collagen in the retina, protecting the eyes against age-related macular degeneration. (AMD).
- Kale, collards and mustard greens. These leafy greens contain high content of vitamin K; they can help slow and ward off cognitive decline, according to new research that reviewed the diets of 1,000 participants. In fact, the researchers discovered that people who ate one or two servings of these greens daily had the cognitive ability of a person 11 years younger than those who consumed none. Kale also contains lutein, a nutrient that reduces the risk of cataracts and age-related macular degeneration, which is the most common cause of blindness among the elderly people.
- Fatty fish. Fish like tuna, wild salmon, mackerel and sardines contain high levels of omega-3 fatty acids, which have been proven to lower overall mortality risk by up to 27 percent and decrease the odds of dying from heart disease by about 35 percent. Eating a few servings of fatty fish each week have been shown to help guard against Alzheimer's disease and help reduce joint pain and stiffness by suppressing the production of enzymes that erode the cartilage. A Harvard School of Public Health study showed that older people with the highest levels

in their blood lived 2.2 years longer on average than those with lower levels of omega-3 fatty acids in their blood. According to research from Ohio State University, a diet abundant in omega-3 fatty acids can preserve the length of telomeres, preventing early aging and premature death.

- Green tea. Okinawa, an island off mainland Japan, is home to more centenarians than anywhere else in the world. They all have one thing in common—deinking green tea every day. Researchers from the Norwich BioScience Institute discovered that the polyphenols, a type of micronutrient in green tea, blocks a compound called VEGF, a signaling molecule in the body that triggers plaque buildup in the arteries that can lead to heart attacks, stroke and vascular disease. The life-extending brew may also ward off wrinkles by fighting inflammation and improving the skin's elasticity, keeping you young both inside and out.

  Researchers from Vanderbilt-Ingram Cancer Center in Nashville

  Found that women who drank green tea at least three times a week lowered their risk of developing cancers of the stomach and esophagus by 17%.

- Tomatoes. Research has found that the reason melanoma rates are so low in regions like Mediterranean—where going topless on the beach is common fun—has to do with the Mediterranean diet, which contains food high in antioxidants, especially deeply colored fruits and vegetables. They seem to help fight the oxidizing effects of harmful ultraviolet rays. One study in the British Journal of Dermatology found participants who ate five tablespoons of tomato paste daily showed 33 percent more protection against sunburn than a control group.

While the carotenoids and antioxidants help the body fight off oxidative stress that ages skin cells, they also boost pro-collagen---a molecule that gives skin its taut, youthful structure.

- Apples. A medium-sized apple is packed with four grams of fiber, which is important for colon health and blood sugar. Apples also contain quercetin, a compound that has been shown to keep arthritis and its associated pain at bay. In a study published in the Journal of Alzheimer's Disease, researchers found that drinking two glasses of apple juice per day is associated the breakup of plaques in the brain that can lead to dementia.

- Mushrooms. They are one of the most health-promoting foods on earth. They contain certain chemical compounds that block the production of estrogen, making them beneficial for breast cancer prevention. Mushrooms also have powerful anti-inflammatory and antioxidant properties, stimulating the immune system, preventing DNA damages and slowing down cancer growth by inhibiting angiogenesis. One caveat: only eat mushrooms cooked because raw mushrooms contain a potentially carcinogenic substance called agaritine that is significantly reduced by cooking.

  One particular mushroom, Shiitaki mushrooms, may have anti-graying property for your aging hair. One cause of early graying is the lack of copper. A study in the journal of Biological Trace Elemental Research found that prematurely graying individuals had significantly lower copper levels than a control group. Your body needs copper to produce pigment for your skin and hair, and shiitaki mushrooms are one of the best dietary sources.

- Nuts. Nuts like walnuts, pistachios, almonds and cashews are high-nutrient sources of healthy fats, plant protein, fiber, minerals, antioxidants and phytosterols. Some may be a little high in calories, but their consumption is associated with lower body weight due to their filling, slowly-digested protein and fiber. They are a low-glycemic food that also helps to reduce the glycemic load of aa entire meal. Eating them regularly can also reduce cholesterol and is linked to a 35 percent reduction in the risk of heart disease. A study published in BioMed Centra showed that people who eat nuts have a 39 percent lower risk of early death than people who don't—and walnut eaters, in particular, have a 45 percent lower risk of dying early.

- Onions, leeks, garlic and scallions. They are known to boost the immune system, protect cardiovascular health, and possess anti-cancer and anti-diabetic effects. Researchers have found that increased consumption of these vegetables is linked to a decrease in the risk of gastric and prostate cancers. Quercetin a flavonoid in onion suppresses tumor growth and proliferation and induces cell death of colon cancer. According to researchers at King's College in London, women who ate garlic and other vegetables in the allium family had a lower risk of osteoarthritis.

- Probiotic yogurt. Among its many health benefits, they contain the probiotic organisms that serve as reinforcements to the good bacteria in your body. They help boost immune system and offer protection against cancer. It also helps to restore the balance to the gastrointestinal tract.

- Oysters. Scientists have shown that these slimy shellfish can help ward off age-related muscle loss and protect your eyes with their protein. They are also a great source of zinc. This mineral helps convert vitamin A, a vital nutrient for the eyes, into a usable form and transport it through blood, slowing the progression of age-related macular degeneration.

- Legumes (beans). They will help you feel full because beans have a stabilizing effect on blood sugar. The soluble fiber lowers your cholesterol levels. Eating at least twice a week has been found to lower colon cancer risk by 50 percent as well as offering significant protection oral, laryngeal, stomach and kidney cancers. Legumes are a good source of protein (plant-based amino acids); as you age, your need for protein will increase. Beans will provide you with fat-free protein along with their disease-fighting fiber and phytochemicals.

- Pomegranate. It is a unique fruit with many health benefits; its signature phytochemical, punicalagin, is the most abundant and is responsible for most of the antioxidant activity of this fruit. The phytochemicals have anti-cancer, cardio-protective and brain-healthy actions, according to many researches. Most notably, a study of patients with severe carotid artery blockages who drank one ounce of pomegranate juice daily for one year, found a 30 percent reduction in atherosclerotic plaque.

- Coffee. It is loaded with antioxidants which can protect against cell damage and lower your risk of chronic diseases including diabetes, heart disease and stroke. A 2012 study in the New England Journal of Medicine showed that coffee drinkers had significantly lower odds of dying during the 13-year study period than did the nob-coffee drinkers. Of course, the coffee should be black without added sugar or creamer.

- Avocado. This fruit is loaded with heart-healthy fats. It is also a great source of glutathione, an antioxidant with strong anti-inflammatory properties.

- Asparagus. It is a natural diuretic and high in potassium and some B-vitamins, important for cell repair and function. Research by scientists at the University of Sydney in Australia showed that B-12 can boost the auditory function. People with lower levels of B-12 have a 33% increased risk of hearing loss.
- Dark chocolate. It is rich in flavonoids, known to decrease blood pressure and levels of cholesterol. British Medical Journal reported that daily consumption of dark chocolate with at least 60 percent cocoa may reduce heart attacks and strokes in high-risk individuals.
- Sweet potatoes. They have high contents of vitamin B-6 and potassium to help protect the immune system and regulate the blood pressure. When eaten with the skin, you get an extra bonus with their generous fiber and beta-carotene.
- Basil and Mint. They have been used for thousands of years in Chinese Medicine to aid digestion and decrease inflammation. Basil and Mint are great sources of luteolin, which can boost the immune system. In 2010, the Journal of Nutrition reported luteolin may even improve memory.
- Olives and olive oil. They are key ingredients in the Mediterranean diet. They are known to lower blood pressure and levels of cholesterol. A new study from the American Academy of Neurology found that olive oil may reduce the risk of stroke too. People 50 or older who regularly used it for cooking and on foods had a 40% lower risk of strokes compared with those who never used it.

There are other world-recognized foods that are healthy and can prolong life expectancy such as bananas, carrots and strawberries. The more we worry about nutrition, the less healthy we seem to become. You don't have to be a scientist or a specialist to know how to eat. Majority of your diets should be plant-based. Simplify your approach with common sense and old-fashioned wisdom.

It is no secret that what you eat has the potential to help you or harm you. Our addiction to processed foods including meat and sugar have left us consuming a diet that offers insufficient nourishment and is the cause of many illnesses we are facing such as obesity, cardiovascular disease, cancer and type two diabetes. It does not have to be this way.

There are many foods, in our country of the plentiful and free, that can leave you feeling energized, reduce your risk of illnesses, allow you to maintain a healthy weight, and offer you a meaningful and productive life.

If you want to live longer and be healthier, you have to fuel your body with the most nutrient-dense foods available. Making natural plant foods a primary part of your diet will restore your health and vitality with longevity.

CHAPTER SEVEN

Aging and Supplements

Getting adequate nutrition can be a challenge as you become older because your body will be less efficient absorbing some key nutrients. Om addition, the ability to taste the food declines, blunting the appetite. Some may have ill-fitting dentures which make chewing and digesting food more difficult. If you live alone as an elderly person, like many seniors do, your diminished appetite for food will not motivate you to make a balanced meal which requires some planning.

Supplementation with vitamins and minerals is a multi-billion dollar industry. About 40 percent of adults age 65 and above take daily vitamins and mineral supplements. According to experts at Emory University, only a fraction of them actually need them. Many ' experts ' asserted that the majority of older people can improve their diet and get the needed nutrients. Realistically, this is easier said than done, when considering other factors surrounding the aging process.

Whether you need supplements or not has been the topic of academic debate for many years, but it is undeniable that the best way to get needed nutrients is to start a well-balanced diet. You may include supplements of vitamins and minerals when there is evidence of limitation of intake, or reduced bodily absorption. It must be emphasized that supplements are not a substitute for a healthy, balanced diet. As you get older, you can become deficient in certain vitamins and minerals and the nutrients you get from your diet alone may not be enough.

Supplements do not cure the aging process!

The most commonly used dietary supplements are the multivitamins. One study of older women suggest multivitamins may not be as helpful as people think. In the study, researchers found an increased risk of death in older women taking several commonly used multivitamins daily.

As a precautionary measure, before starting any vitamin/mineral supplements, you should consult your doctor or nutritionist/dietician to determine if it is appropriate and necessary. Because some supplements may affect the way prescription drugs work. As a consumer, do your due diligence and be prudent and judicious about their uses.

What are vitamins and minerals?

Vitamins are micro-nutrients that your body needs in small amounts to stay healthy. The amount you needed depends on the vitamins. Because your body can only make limited amounts of vitamins for itself, the rest should come from a nutritious, balanced diet. Minerals are also micro-nutrients your body needs to function properly. Examples of minerals include iron, calcium, zinc, magnesium and selenium. Anyway, supplements should not be taken or started blindly without assessing the food intake history of older adults, in particular.

Vitamin D

Let us start with the ever-popular vitamin D. One study in 2012 found that 40 percent of the U.S. adults were deficient in vitamin D, and one in five UK adults have low levels of vitamin D. At least one billion people worldwide are not getting enough vitamin D, according to the Harvard School of Public Health, especially those that live north of the northern hemisphere during winter and spring, with latitudinal lines connecting San Francisco to Philadelphia or Athens to Beijing. Here, the sun's rays are just not strong enough, and it is almost impossible for anyone to satisfy vitamin D needs through diet alone. It is my opinion that it really requires a three-pronged approach: sun exposure, supplements and foods.

Doctors have long routinely advised older patients who are more likely to have low vitamin D levels too increase their intake through supplementation. The Endocrine Society recommends consuming at 1,500 to 2,000 IU of vitamin D daily.

There are two forms of vitamin D: D2 and D3. D3 (cholecalciferol) is the form of vitamin D actively made by and used in the body. Normally, vitamin D is made when you go outside and your skin gets exposed to the sun. As you get older, you might not get enough sunlight, especially in the winter. Also, your skin and other organs that are responsible for making vitamin D might not work as well with the aging process. Simply put, there is a definite decrease in the way the skin makes vitamin D.

Since vitamin D is such an important vitamin crucial for your overall wellbeing; it is essential for building bone and maintaining skeletal structure, promoting calcium absorption, aiding immune function and helping to reduce inflammation. Let us look at some of the hints, symptoms and signs that you may not be getting enough of this vital vitamin:

- Feeling bloated and constipated with abdominal pain and alternating diarrhea is associated with irritable bowel syndrome (IBS). According to a study in BMJ Open Gastroenterology, over 75 percent of people with IBS had low levels of vitamin D.
- Poor athletic performance despite your enthusiasm and physical training. Low levels of vitamin D increase inflammation and slows speed of recovery from intense exercise.
- You are tired all the time with unexpected weakness, even though you have enough sleep and normal levels of iron.
- You have aches and pain in muscles and bones, especially in the winter, with stiffness.
- Sweaty forehead. An excessively sweaty forehead without strenuous exercise and while your activity level remains steady and you are in a moderate temperature environment.
- Erectile dysfunction. Men with ED often have cardiovascular disease, which is associated with vitamin D deficiency.
- You are prone to stress fractures. You need vitamin D to absorb calcium properly for bone health.
- You might have problem with insomnia.
- You are catching colds and flu more easily. Low levels of vitamin D can result in depressed immune system.
- You are feeling depressed. Vitamin D seems to have the same effects as the feel-good hormones, like serotonin, even though the exact mechanism is still unknown. There are receptors for vitamin D in many parts of the brain.

Of course, a blood test for your vitamin D level is really the only way to accurately determine whether you have a vitamin D deficiency or not.

There are many health benefits that are linked to sufficient and therapeutic high levels of vitamin D, but links don't necessarily prove cause and effect. There can be many other explanations for the associations observed. Several large-scale randomized trials of vitamin D are in progress, and they will hopefully provide conclusive evidence as to whether supplementations with moderate to high doses of vitamin C can reduce the risk of heart disease, cancer, and other chronic illnesses.

In the meantime, let us look at some of the health benefits that vitamin D may play a role:

Multiple Sclerosis—In 2013, an international team of researchers examined data from 465 people with early-stage multiple sclerosis (MS). A disabling autoimmune disease that affects the central nervous system. They reported that people with high levels of 25-hydroxy D had a slower rate of disease progression with fewer new brain lesions, lower brain volume loss and lower disability levels than those with low levels of vitamin D.

Pre-menstrual syndrome—According to the Nurses' Health Study II, women between the ages of 27 and 44 with a high intake of vitamin D had the lowest risk of experiencing PMS symptoms. The study also found that higher calcium intake was associated with lower PMS symptoms also. Sometimes, pre-eclampsia occurs during pregnancy, and this can cause the expecting mother to have elevated blood pressure. Eclampsia is characterized by onset of seizures in women who have pre-eclampsia. Studied have found that normal, pregnant women generally have higher levels of vitamin D than women who suffer pre-eclampsia and eclampsia.

Dental health—The sunshine vitamin has a key role in protecting your teeth as you age. In one study, older adults who took 700 international units (IU) of vitamin D, along with calcium each day for three years were less likely to lose teeth than those who took placebo pills, even two years after they stopped taking the supplements.

Dementia—In a recent study in JAMA Neurology, which measured vitamin D and cognitive function each year in an ethnically diverse group of elderly patients (about half of whom had some form of cognitive impairment at the start of the study), lower levels of D were associated with accelerated cognitive decline. According to the VITAL study at Harvard University, older people with vitamin D deficiency performed poorly on tests of memory, attention and reasoning compared to people with adequate levels of vitamin D in their blood.

Many clinical studies have shown that vitamin D helps with brain function, probably by strengthening the neural circuits. Low levels of this vitamin have been found in patients living with Alzheimer's, multiple sclerosis and Parkinson's, but it is currently inconclusive or unclear whether or not vitamin D can help treat or prevent these neuro-degenerative diseases. But, what do you have to lose if you are suffering from these ' incurable ' illnesses?

Depression—Female college students who had low levels of vitamin D were more likely to have clinically significant symptoms of depression, according to a 2015 study published in Psychiatry Research. A large meta-analysis of more than 31,000 research subjects, published in the British Journal of Psychiatry, found a correlation as well. So, correcting the deficiency of vitamin D can make the elderly people a lot happier. This does not necessarily mean that vitamin D deficiency causes depression, but it is clear that vitamin D supports brain health, in general.

Colorectal cancer—A 2011 meta-analysis that included more than one million study subjects found that higher vitamin D intake and higher vitamin D levels were linked to lower risk of colorectal cancer.

Breast cancer. Some studies have suggested that there may be a link between higher levels of vitamin D and a lowered risk of breast cancer, especially post-menopausal women.

Pancreatic cancer—People with the highest vitamin D levels were 35 percent less likely to develop pancreatic cancer than those with the lowest levels, according to a20-year of nearly 120,000 people conducted by researchers from Brigham and Women's Hospital in Massachusetts.

Prostate cancer—Low levels of vitamin D were associated with more advanced, aggressive prostate tumors in biopsy patients in a 2014 study in Clinical Cancer Research; among African Americans, low levels of vitamin D was also associated with a higher risk of developing prostate cancer in the first place. A small pilot study from the Medical University of South Carolina in Charleston found that when patients with prostate cancers received 4,000 IU of vitamin D per day for 60 days, 60% of them showed improvement in their tumors.

Diabetes—People with diabetes or prediabetes have lower vitamin D levels than those with normal blood sugar, according to a Spanish study published in 2015 in the journal of Clinical Endocrinology and Metabolism. Studies have shown that vitamin D seems to improve insulin sensitivity, and decrease insulin resistance which leads to sugar buildup in the blood.

Heart disease—Heart disease and vitamin D deficiency are known to go hand in hand. Many studies have shown that subjects with very low levels of vitamin D were nearly three times as likely to die of heart failure and five times as likely to die of sudden cardiac death. Make sure you have sufficient vitamin D in your body for a long life span.

Osteoporosis—With age, our bones tend to shrink in size and density. Our bodies need vitamin D to help absorb calcium and grow bones that stay dense and strong throughout your life. Older women can improve their bone health significantly with vitamin D and calcium supplements along with exercise.

Female incontinence—Since vitamin D is important for muscle strength, deficiency can cause weakness in the pelvic floor and lead to urinary incontinence. The pelvic floor is a hammock of muscles that supports the bladder, uterus and rectum. In fact, a weak pelvic floor can also lead to fecal incontinence, according to a 2012 research review published in International Urogynecology Journal. For older women who suffer from poor bladder control, maintaining healthy levels of vitamin D can prove to be as important as performing pelvic floor exercises.

Improving physical performance—Low levels of vitamin D can seriously hinder your strength and athletic performance, according to a recent study from the University of Tulsa. One theory is that vitamin D may help your muscle cells release calcium more efficiently during the muscle contraction process. This can lead to faster and more powerful contractions, resulting in higher jump, faster sprint and heavier lift.

Immune system function—Many studies have shown that vitamin D helps your immune system fend off viruses and bacteria. A 2017 analysis found that vitamin D reduced the risk of respiratory infections when taken daily or every other day in supplement form. There have been many studies looking at the connections between vitamin D and COVID-19 infections. There is no clinical evidence to prove low levels of vitamin D leading to severe Covid-19 symptoms, but there is definite a linkage between the sunshine vitamin and immune responses to the disease with abundant data to support a large beneficial effect. According to most experts, the preponderance of evidence indicates that increased vitamin D would help reduce infections, hospitalizations, ICU admissions and deaths caused by COVID-19.

Longer life span. Women who spent the most time in the sun outlived those who avoided its rays, according to a recent study that followed almost 30,000 Swedish women for 20 years, taking smoking, exercise and obesity into consideration. The possible explanation is the boost in vitamin D study participants get could improve their cardiovascular health.

There are many sources of vitamin D, and the cheapest one is going outside. Vitamin D is created when the ultraviolet B rays of the sun hit the skin. Sitting outside for as little as 10 minutes is sufficient for most people. Many other outdoor activities such as gardening, biking and playing sports are just as effective. Be sure to take sun-safety precautions for extended periods spent out in the sun due to the increased risk of developing skin cancer.

The sources of vitamin D from food are so great and common, it is ironic that deficiency of vitamin D is fairly common in this world. Here is a list of common foods that can provide you with dietary vitamin D:

- Fatty fish such as sardines, salmon and canned tuna
- Eel
- Egg yolks
- Beef liver
- Red meat
- Cod liver oil
- Fortified milk
- Fortified breakfast cereals
- Mushrooms
- Fortified orange juice
- Tofu
- Caviar
- Pork, such as lean ham
- Ricotta cheese
- Oatmeal
- Dried prunes—rich in vitamin D and Calcium

Is it possible to take too much vitamin D in the form of supplement? The answer is ' yes '. It is important to take only the recommended dose under the supervision of your physician because vitamin D is not water-soluble, but it is fat-soluble, meaning its levels can accumulate in your body and become toxic. Some of the symptoms of vitamin D toxicity and poisoning include kidney stones, bone pain, muscle weakness, nausea and vomiting.

Vitamin B-12, the energy vitamin

About 10 to 15 percent of adults have B-12 deficiency. It develops slowly and is more common with older people. Since the symptoms are similar to many other conditions associated with aging, it is sometimes overlooked.

B-12 deficiency can occur due to diet. But, most often a deficiency occurs when the body does not digest and absorb B-12. Causes can be changes due to aging, celiac disease, Crohn's disease or prolonged use of antacids, over-the-counter acid blockers, or prescription medications used to treat gastroesophageal reflux and heartburn. Acid in the stomach is needed for B-12 to detach it from its original protein so it can be absorbed into the bloodstream. When you are over 50, it is normal for the body to produce less gastric acid, making older people prone to B-12 deficiency.

A study from England found that out of 283 type 2 diabetics on high-dose metformin, 33 percent had a vitamin B-12 deficiency. This does not mean that all diabetics will have a vitamin B-12 problem.

Heavy drinking can cause gastritis or irritation of the stomach lining, and this can lead to low stomach acid and lead to decreased B-12 absorption. B-12 is stored in the liver, and alcohol consumption can impair liver function and deplete B-12 stores or make it harder for the liver to use it.

B-12 deficiency is linked to pernicious anemia. It is a deficiency of red blood cells that happens when the stomach does not produce enough of a protein called intrinsic factor, which helps intestine absorb B-12. In this case of anemia, the body produces large, immature red blood cells that can't carry oxygen throughout the body; thus, leading to pale, yellowish skin without that healthy glow.

Intrinsic factor is needed for the intestines to absorb B-12. But some data suggest that intrinsic factor is not necessarily needed if B-12 supplementation is high enough and that B-12 gets absorbed by a passive mechanism when its stomach concentration is high enough.

B-12 is a powerhouse. It helps make DNA, nerve and blood cells, and is crucial for a healthy brain and immune system. Its deficiency can cause memory loss, disorientation and difficulty thinking and reasoning, and thus can be mistaken for dementia. Experts advised that people with unexplained cognitive decline should be tested for B-12 deficiency since B-12 works closely with the metabolic processes in the brain. If the cognitive decline is related to diet and B-12 deficiency, then that is easily correctable. Sometimes, severe vitamin B12 deficiency, also known as pernicious anemia, is misdiagnosed as dementia because signs and symptoms of B12 deficiency include depression, memory loss, impaired cognitive function and peripheral neuropathy.

Rush University Medical Center in Chicago studied 121 people age 65 or older who had signs of a B-12 deficiency. Researchers followed up four and a half years later and found that participants who exhibited four out of five signs of a B-12 deficiency were at a higher risk for getting low cognitive test scores and smaller brain volumes.

B-12 is crucial for the making for myelin of the central nervous system (the brain and the spinal cord). A deficiency of B-12 can cause your hands feeling numb and tingling, a pin-and-needle sensation. In fact, many studies have shown that low B12 level is an important risk factor for loss of brain volume among older people, and the serum B12 status may be an early marker of brain atrophy, according to neuroscientific research.

Vitamin B-12 helps boost the production of neurotransmitters and communication between nerves, so a shortage of B-12 can lead to a shortage of serotonin, making you more prone to depression. Serotonin is a neurotransmitter that keeps your brain and mood functioning correctly.

Vitamin B-12 also plays an important role in the production of white blood cells, which are essential for proper functioning of your immune system. However, the absorption of B-12 can be a problem, often unnoticed, for the geriatric group with decreased gastric acid production. Many of them are taking either OTC antacids and/or prescriptions for proton pump inhibitors such as Nexium and Prilosec for conditions like reflux esophagitis, dyspepsia and peptic ulcer disease. This low gastric acid environment, iatrogenic, and the subsequent decrease in vitamin-12 absorption can be exacerbated by the tendency of the senior population to consume fewer foods that are rich in vitamin B-12 such as red meat (grass-fed), and shellfish (oysters, clams, mussels, shrimp and scallops). Many of them living on their own with limited budgets are more likely to choose convenient and cheaper carbohydrates such as bread, noodles, pasta and spaghetti which are easier to prepare and chew, rather than cooking a meal of healthy fat and proteins for themselves.

Plants don't make vitamin B-12. It is only found in animal products like eggs, meat, shellfish, poultry and dairy products. Strict vegetarians are at high risk for developing a B-12 deficiency if they do not eat grains that have been fortified with the vitamin B-12 or take a B-12 supplement.

Magnesium

It is a chemical element with a symbol Mg. Its absorption decreases with age. Its levels in the body can also be reduced by pharmaceutical

medications like diuretics which many older people take for various health issues. Magnesium can be lost from your body also with the use of alcohol, coffee, black tea, soy and calcium supplements.

Even with a balanced diet, you may still have insufficient levels of magnesium in your body. I personally suggest that just meeting the daily requirement is not ideal; try to have the optimum levels of this essential mineral that is necessary for good health and is a vital component within our cells. It provides protection from many chronic diseases, especially those associated with aging and stress. In fact, many medical researchers have suggested at least doubling the current recommendations due to its many health benefits.

Here are some of the health benefits of this ancient nutrient:

- Better sleep. Melatonin, the sleep regulating hormone, is disturbed when you are deficient in magnesium. Magnesium helps regulate the balance and control stress hormones, decreasing your stress and tension for better sleep.
- Mood elevator. Magnesium acts as a precursor for serotonin, increasing the production of the neurotransmitter, serotonin, which relaxes the Central Nervous System and improves your mood. It may help your depression according to the National Institute of Health.

- Growth and strength of muscles. Magnesium promotes the production of Growth Hormone (IGF-1) for the muscles. Furthermore, adenosine triphosphate (ATP) is the cell's energy store, and Magnesium helps boost ATP levels by activating it.

- Relieving muscle cramp. Low levels of Magnesium can lead to buildup of lactic acid, resulting in muscle cramps and tightness. So, it is good for flexibility of muscles and decrease of post-workout muscle aches.

- Bone health. Calcium is not the only nutrient for your bones, there are at least fifteen more essential elements that contribute to bone health; magnesium is one of the most essential and important ones. Magnesium stimulates a particular hormone, called Calcitonin, which suppresses the parathyroid hormone. Too much parathyroid hormone leads to osteolytic activities (breakdown) in the bones.

- Enzymatic functions. Magnesium is needed for many biochemical reactions in the body. For example, it acts as a co-enzyme in the digestive tract, aiding in the breakdown of foods and assimilation of nutrients into our bodies.

- Anti-diabetic effect. Magnesium enhances insulin secretion and facilitates the transfer of glucose into the cells. In other words, it helps regulating healthy blood sugar levels. Magnesium deficiency can lead to insulin resistance.

- Heart health. Magnesium helps to maintain a healthy heart, as it aids in the proper transfer of potassium, calcium and other nutrient ions across the cell membranes. According to a 2006 study published in the journal Modern Nutrition in Health and Disease, these nutrients are important to promote healthy nerve impulses, muscle contractions and normal cardiac rhythm. Few of us drink hard water anymore, thanks to the water purification and softening processes. This process removes some minerals including iron, magnesium and calcium found in hard water. According to a report by the World Health Organization, native communities who consume hard water showed fewer problems with cardiovascular disease when compared to natives who moved into more urban settings.

One study by the Honolulu Heart Program of 1,000 men taking magnesium supplements; the researchers found that those who took more than the daily recommended intake of 400 mg developed fewer heart problems than those who took less than 320 mg of magnesium.

- Cellular synthesis. As one of its many biochemical functions, Magnesium serves as a building block for RNA and DNA synthesis.

- A powerful detoxifier. Heavy metals, pesticides, herbicides and many other environmental harmful chemicals and toxins are greatly inhibited from accumulating when Magnesium is present in sufficient concentration.

- Reduction of cancer risk. A recent study published in the American Journal of Clinical Nutrition found that for every 100-mg increase in Magnesium intake, a person's risk of developing colorectal cancer drops by 13 percent. Magnesium has anti-inflammatory properties, and we know that inflammation is shown to be a leading cause of many diseases, including cancer. A meta-analysis by the International Society for the Development of Research on Magnesium found that low levels of this mineral negatively affect the permeability of cells, which has been shown to initiate carcinogenesis.

There are many forms of Magnesium being sold on the market as supplements. The substance used in any given supplement compound can affect the absorption and bioavailability of Magnesium. The more common ones include magnesium oxide, magnesium sulfate, magnesium hydroxide and magnesium citrate. You need to consult your physician regarding your choices. One thing they have in common: the laxative properties.

Few people get enough Magnesium in their diets these days. In fact, calcium tends to be over-utilized and taken in high quantities. This can cause more harm than good, as it is important to have a proper balance between calcium and magnesium. Whole foods are the best sources for magnesium. Foods high in fiber such as dark leafy greens, nuts, seeds like pumpkin, beans, avocados and bananas are great sources. Kelp, a type of seaweed, is also a rich source of magnesium.

Calcium

Almost all the calcium in your body is found in your bones. As you age, calcium tends to leave your bones which can put you at risk for osteoporosis. Calcium deficiency may also put you at risk for osteomalacia, which is softening pf the bones.

If you don't like dairy products, you probably should consider calcium supplements, since the ideal source of calcium is dairy products. Because vitamin D helps you absorb more calcium, you may need to take both vitamin D and calcium supplements at the same time.

Several forms of calcium supplements are available in the stores known as calcium salts. Each calcium salt has different amount of calcium in it. For example, calcium carbonate has more calcium in it than calcium citrate.

When taking calcium supplements, you might experience constipation. You can decrease this side effect by drinking plenty of fluid, eating lots of fiber and exercising.

Let us look at some of the foods that are rich in calcium and can help strengthen your bones:

- Dark leafy greens such as bok choy, kale, collard greens and broccoli. They are a good source of calcium; along with the potassium, they can help reduce your risk of osteoporosis.
- Figs, dried or fresh, are loaded with calcium, potassium and magnesium; they are definitely bone builders.
- Salmon is a good source of calcium, in addition to its heart-healthy omega-3 fatty acids.
- Almond butter provides an easy way to boost your calcium intake. Moreover, almond has potassium, protein and other nutrients that play a supportive role in building strong bones.
- Tofu is rich in calcium and protein, and is ideal for older people because it is easy to digest and swallowed.
- Dried prunes are excellent sources of calcium and vitamin D, which can help improve your bone density.

Special note: Smoothies made with yogurt, fruits and vegetables can be excellent source of calcium along with many other nutrients for older people who have decreased appetite, have trouble chewing or have a dry mouth.

Omega-3 fatty acids

We just can't say enough about these wonderful heart-healthy fats these days. These unsaturated fats have many health benefits including alleviating some of the symptoms of rheumatoid arthritis, slowing the progression of age-related macular degeneration (the most common cause of vision loss among seniors), lowering the risk of Alzheimer's disease and perhaps even keeping your brain sharper as you age, and protecting your heart.

Omega-3 fatty acids can be found in foods such as nuts, beans and seeds besides fatty fish, but fish are the most ideal sources for older people. Seniors should have at least two servings of fish a week with salmon, tuna, mackerel or sardine. Preparing the ingredients to make a fish dinner can be challenging for some seniors; they can make it easy for themselves just adding some canned salmon or tuna on their salads without losing out on the omega-3 fatty acids.

Vitamin C

No discussion of vitamin supplements can go on without including vitamin C. It is such a famous micro-nutrient with believers and skeptics for its many health benefits. There has always been a concern about over-utilization of vitamin C, and some people claimed that a healthy diet rich in fruit and vegetable should provide sufficient levels of vitamin C. This may be true for younger people who follow a plant-based diet. Studies have shown that older adults have higher requirements for vitamin C.

The body neither makes nor stores vitamin C, and you must eat foods containing this vitamin every day. A vitamin C intake of at least 400mg daily may be particularly important for older adults who are at higher risk for age-related chronic diseases. As one of the many antioxidants, vitamin C reduces free radicals, the damaging chemicals responsible for aging. It protects against oxidative stress to cells and biological molecules.

Vitamin C is an integral part of many structures of our body; it plays an important role in building and repairing tissues such as skin, blood vessels, tendons and ligaments, bones, teeth and cartilage. The body cannot make collagen without vitamin C working as a co-factor, and it would fall apart without the protein collagen.

Scurvy is no longer a familiar sight, but once a scourge, devastating the lives of sailors, who were deprived of fresh foods including vegetables on their long voyages. These afflicted individuals suffered weakened limbs, which became swollen and discolored while their gums bled profusely. Other symptoms included easy bruising, anemia, fatigue, heart failure and eventually death.

Vitamin C may help those with immune system weakened by stress, may reduce the risk of stroke, reduces complications from colds and flu, and improves skin health. These benefits to the body were discovered by researcher at the University of Michigan based on information from more than 100 studies of vitamin C over a 10-year period.

A study also found that women between the ages of 40 and 74 with high levels of vitamin C experienced fewer problems with dry skin and fewer wrinkles.

Evidence suggests that people with high levels of vitamin C from fruits and vegetables may experience a lower risk of getting certain cancers, according to the National Institute of Health Office of Dietary Supplements. These cancers include breast, colon and lung.

Vitamin C can also benefit the body when one smokes, is an alcoholic or obese because these conditions cause the levels of vitamin C to drop.

The bodies of smokers, in particular, need vitamin C because of the considerable amounts of free radicals generated by cigarette smoking.

The dosages of vitamin C, especially at high levels, are controversial. It probably varies among different individuals with different stress levels, lifestyle habits and health conditions. Even though it is water soluble and your body does not store it, side effects can still occur, such as stomach pain, diarrhea and flatulence at excessively high doses. If you take prescription medications, ask your doctor if it is safe to take vitamin C above the recommendations. Vitamin C, at massive doses, can interact with medications such as aspirin, antacids and blood thinners.

Niacin

Dietary surveys indicate that 15% to 25% pf older adults do not consume enough niacin in their diets, and that dietary intake of niacin decrease between the ages of 60 and 90 years. Thus, it is advisable for older adults to supplement their diet with a daily multivitamin which will generally provide at least 20mg of niacin.

Niacin is one of the eight B vitamins, called B-3; it is one of the essential human nutrients. It causes the blood vessels to dilate or open up near the skin shortly after taking it, resulting in the notorious niacin flush, a hot, tingling sensation accompanied by a red, flushing of the skin. This reaction is not dangerous and is transient, just uncomfortable for some people. Tolerance will occur over time and the flush will get less and less noticeable.

Like other B vitamins, niacin helps the body break down carbohydrates, fats and proteins into energy. Let us look at some of the known health benefits with niacin:

- Relief of arthritis symptoms. Several studies have reported excellent results for alleviation of some of the arthritis symptoms with dosages ranging from 1,000 to 1,500mg a day in divided doses.

- Decrease of cholesterol and triglyceride. Researchers found that participants taking between 1,000 and 2,000mg of niacin a day showed at least 25 percent reduction of cholesterol and triglyceride levels.

- Heart benefit. Heart patients receiving niacin have lower death rates after 5 years when compared to those not using niacin, according to Nutritional research. This is primarily due to the reduction of VLDL, cholesterol and triglyceride, and improvement of circulation from dilation of blood vessels.

- Brain health. Dr. Abram Hoffer, famous for his use of niacin in the treatment of schizophrenia and depression, has reported that 1,000mg of niacin, two to three times a day can improve memory and some senility problems.

- Erectile dysfunction. Some studies have shown that patients suffering from erectile dysfunction and dyslipidemia (cholesterol and triglyceride abnormalities) reported significant improvement of ED while receiving 1,500mg of niacin for twelve weeks.

- Insomnia. Niacinamide activates the benzodiazepine receptors in the brain, resulting in sedation. So, taking 250mg to 500mg of niacin can help alleviate some of your insomnia problems.

- Stroke benefit. Some studies have found that taking niacin may help stroke patients. When rats with ischemic stroke were given niacin, their brains grew new blood vessels, according to researchers at Henry Ford Hospital in Detroit, Michigan. Ischemic stroke is caused by an obstruction within a blood vessel supplying blood to the brain and accounts for 87 percent of all stroke cases. Another study in 2000 published in the journal Stroke also used rats and found that treatment with niacinamide may repair damage to the brain caused by strokes.
- Acne. In a double-blind trials by the State University of New York, the topical application of a 4% niacinamide, twice a day for two months resulted in a similar acne improvement when compared to 1% clindamycin gel. Of course, we are not concerned about acne among the older adults.

Like anything else, moderation is the key, and you will need to know how much your body can handle the amount of supplements. Supplements, like medications, have their known side effects. Niacin can cause gastric irritation if taken on an empty stomach. If you have gouty arthritis, be aware that niacin may compete with the excretion of uric acid precipitating a gouty attack. Moreover, the slow-release form has been shown to cause some liver damage. It is prudent and safe practice to check with your physician if you are planning on supplementing your body with niacin above the recommended levels.

Zinc

Zinc is a naturally occurring mineral found in food and is vital to your health. New research published in the British Journal of Nutrition suggests that even a small or short-term zinc deficiency can lead to virtually undetectable damage. According to the World Health Organization, zinc deficiency affects about one third of the world's population, and it is reasonable to presume that zinc deficiency can be a problem for the older adults.

Zinc is involved in the production of at least 30 enzymes, important for many biochemical processes in our bodies, from producing DNA to repairing cells. It is important for proper functioning of the immune and digestive systems, control of diabetes, reduction of stress levels, energy metabolism and increased rate of healing for acne and wounds. It is also important for the sense of smell.

Zinc is also important for men because of its role in maintaining prostate health, testosterone levels and overall sexual health. Since our bodies do not make zinc, a daily intake is necessary to ensure healthy levels of this critical mineral.

The following is a brief summary of what zinc can do for your health:

- The pancreas is the control center for food digestion; it pumps zinc into the gastrointestinal tract in order to maintain a consistent level for digestive enzymes. Decreased zinc level will interrupt the digestive system, causing accumulation of undigested foods inside the GI tract, resulting in loss of appetite because of feeling less hungry.
- Diabetic people typically have lower zinc levels when compared with healthy, non-diabetic people. According to some studies, zinc supplementation may improve blood sugar control in type-2 diabetics.

- Scientists at Wayne State University School of Medicine found that young men who restricted dietary zinc intake for 20 weeks saw decreases in testosterone levels, while zinc-deficient elderly men taking zinc supplements for six months experienced increases in testosterone production. They also discovered that older men who don't have sufficient levels of zinc in their diets tend to have higher instances of enlarged prostate, called benign prostatic hypertrophy (BPH) and prostatitis. They also have a higher rate of prostate cancer.

- Boosting the immune system. Zinc became a popular cold remedy when a 1996 report published by Cleveland Clinic said that zinc could help reduce a cold's severity and duration. A study of 100 people who had cold symptoms for less than 24 hours took zinc lozenges every two hours; half took a placebo. The zinc users reported that their cold symptoms lasted an average of 4.4 days, compared with 7.6 days for those who used a placebo.

- Baldness. According to a study in Australia, men who ate lean meat (a rich source of zinc) were less likely to go bald than those who consumed fatty cuts of meat. Thus, not getting enough zinc can lead to hair loss.

- Alcoholic consumption can lower the levels of zinc in the body, causing alcohol-induced liver damage. Alcoholics who took zinc supplement experienced less live damage because zinc promotes the enzymes that help dissipate alcohol.

- Disease fighting. Zinc helps to increase the production of white blood cells that fight infections. It also increases the number of killer cells that fight against cancer and aids in the release of antibodies form the white blood cells. The elderly people who are often deficient in zinc with a weaker immune system due to age; zinc supplements may increase the number of infection-fighting T-cells and boost the immune system.

- Skin health. Zinc can help acne blemishes heal faster, reduce inflammation caused by acne and aid in regulating skin's oil gland activity affected by changing hormones.
- Thyroid health. Zinc is a key mineral that helps produce the thyroid releasing hormone (TRH) in your brain, which then signal the pituitary gland to make thyroid stimulating hormone (TSH). According to several studies, low zinc levels are associated with low T-3 (the active thyroid hormone) and a reduced ability to convert T-4 to T-3.

There are many sources of zinc from food, but animal foods are better than plant foods in terms of zinc contents with oysters on top of the list:

- Oysters
- Beef
- Lamb
- Crabs
- Lobsters
- Pork
- Chicken
- Dairy products
- Wheat germs
- Spinach
- Pumpkin seeds
- Sesame seeds
- Sunflower seeds
- Flaxseeds
- Cashew nuts

- Pecan
- Almonds
- Walnuts
- Peanut
- Hazelnuts

Co-enzyme Q10

Co-enzyme Q10 is a fat-soluble compound, primarily synthesized in the body. It is a powerful antioxidant, but the body makes less and less of it with age. Studies have shown decreased tissue levels of Co-enzyme Q10 as one gets older. Low levels are also found in people with cancer, diabetes, heart disease, Parkinson's disease and HIV/AIDS.

It is a critical co-factor in our energy production pathways. In both animal and human studies, co-enzyme Q10 can compensate for immune deficiency caused by aging and chronic disease.

According to the Free Radical and Mitochondrial theories of aging, oxidative damage of cell structures by reactive oxygen species (ROS) play an important role in the functional declines that accompanying aging. ROS may damage mitochondria over time, causing them to function less efficiently and to generate more damaging ROS in a self-perpetuating cycle. Co-enzyme Q10, also known as ubiquinone, plays an important role in mitochondrial ATP synthesis and function as an antioxidant in mitochondrial membranes.

CoQ10 has received a lot of attention in the scientific medical community because of its health beneficial potential. Many studies have shown that taking CoQ10 in supplemental form can offer anti-aging benefits.

According to a report published in Pharmacology and Therapeutics in 2009, it may benefit patients with atherosclerosis, heart failure and coronary artery disease.

CoQ10 also shows promise in the treatment of neurodegenerative disorders such as Alzheimer's disease and Parkinson's disease, according to a research review published in Neuropsychiatric Disease and Treatment in 2009. CoQ10 may inhibit overproduction of beta amyloid, a protein fragment that forms the plaques associated with Alzheimer's disease. There is not yet any conclusive evidence to recommend CoQ10 for prevention or treatment of the disease at this time.

Food sources of Co-Q10 include meat, poultry, fish, soybeans and nuts. Fruits, vegetables and dairy products also contain Co-Q10 to some degree.

Thiamin

It is commonly known as B-1, sometimes it is called the anti-stress vitamin because it strengthens the immune system. As part of the eight nutrients that make up the B-Complex family, B-1 plays an important role in brain, nerves, muscle and heart function.

Many studies have found inadequate dietary intake and thiamin deficiency to be more common in the elderly population. Thus it would be prudent and healthy for older adults to take one multivitamin a day as a supplement. One tablet of multivitamin generally provides at least 1.5 mg of thiamin.

Thiamin is water-soluble, and is used by the body for many biochemical reactions. Every cell in the body needs thiamin in order to form ATP. It helps the body to convert food into fuel (glucose) which is then used to produce energy.

It might be beneficial for people with Alzheimer's disease and older adults with mental impairment. A 4-year study found that epileptics taking 50 to 100 mg of thiamin had better mental function and tet scores than those who took a placebo.

Alcoholics often suffer from thiamin deficiency because alcohol makes it difficult for the body to absorb the nutrient from the food. A thiamin supplement of 50 to 100 mg a day is beneficial for people who drink alcohol regularly.

You will find dietary thiamin in foods high in protein like beef, pork, poultry, nuts, eggs, legumes and seeds.

Selenium

It is a trace element and mineral that is essential for human life. It is found naturally in soil. In general, a balanced diet with 80% fruits and vegetables and a multivitamin containing some selenium should be sufficient for its need.

Researchers and nutritional scientists have found some special health benefits with selenium supplementation, especially in the area of anti-aging.

- It is a powerful antioxidant, and can protect against free radicals and oxidative stress, resulting in less cellular damage. One study revealed that selenium levels decline with age and low selenium levels contribute to cognitive decline in older adults. Studies are in progress to determine whether supplementation of selenium can slow age-related mental impairment.

- There is some evidence that supplementing with selenium helps mercury excretion from the body.

- Cardiovascular support. Many studies have shown that there is relationship between selenium and cardiovascular health. Low selenium levels were found in patients with heart failure and heart attack. With its anti-inflammatory and antioxidant properties, it certainly can lend a hand to maintaining heart health.

- Thyroid support. Compared to other tissues in the human body, the thyroid contains the most selenium per gram. Like iodine, selenium plays a vital role in the synthesis of thyroid hormones.

Natural sources like fruits and vegetables are the best way to incorporate selenium into your diet to enjoy its many health benefits. Many studies have shown that selenium is important to your health and longevity. Many chronic illnesses increase as you age, selenium can help defend your body and contribute to a long life!

Vitamin E

Vitamin E has been gaining a lot of attention and popularity like its counter-part, vitamin D. It is a fat-soluble nutrient that can be found in many foods including fruits and vegetables, vegetable oils, cereals, meats, poultry, eggs and wheat germ oil. The National Institute of Health states that vitamin E acts as an antioxidant, helping to protect cells from the damage caused by free radicals.

It is arguably one of the most widely used supplements today, and are sold over the counter in many pharmacies and department stores. It is found naturally in eight different forms and the most important one is the one containing alpha-tocopherol Being fat-soluble, it is stored in the fat cells of the body. When the fat cells are saturated, the excess fat-soluble vitamin is stored in the liver. Vitamin E is an antioxidant working in lipids, and this makes it complementary to vitamin C, which is a powerful antioxidant fighting free radicals in the water.

There have been numerous reports about the health benefits and therapeutic values of vitamin E supplementation; some are considered by skeptics as anecdotal from self-reporting, but many were based on scientific and epidemiologic studies awaiting conclusive evidences. Nonetheless, it is fair to say that we need to deal with this wonderful vitamin with an open mind and informed caution. The American Heart Association, at this time, recommends obtaining vitamin E by eating a well-balanced diet high in fruits, vegetables and whole grains rather than from supplements until more is known about the risks and benefits of taking the supplements.

Let us look at some of the many health benefits of vitamin E, especially for the older adults:

- It can prevent clogging of the arteries that contribute to cardiovascular diseases. Studies have shown that patients with atherosclerosis who take vitamin E supplement showed significantly less plaque buildup in the arteries than those in a control group who were taking a placebo. However, some studies have suggested that excessive supplemental intake of it can increase the risk of bleeding in people on antiplatelet medications.

- Some studies have shown that it may reduce the risk of death from stroke in post-menopausal women.

- According to some research, it may inhibit the growth of malignant cells in cancers associated with hormonal causes, for example, prostate and breast cancers. But, a large study in 2015 of 35,533 men taking vitamin E supplements found that it could increase the risk of prostate cancer for men, but the dosage ranges exceeding the recommendation could not be ascertained.

- It may prevent osteoarthritis, and is useful for pain relief and treatment of inflamed joints due to its anti-inflammatory properties.

- It may improve cognitive performances in patients with Alzheimer's disease, and in conjunction with vitamin C, may prevent the development of Alzheimer's disease, according to some studies.

- It seems to have protective effects against the development of cataracts and age-related macular degeneration.

- According to researchers of some anti-aging studies, vitamin E may slow the effects of aging including the brain.

- There is some evidence that vitamin E can help lower the blood pressure.

- Some studies have shown that it can help control blood sugar and cholesterol levels in people with type-2 diabetes and decrease the cardiovascular complications. Recent research discovers that about 40% of the people with diabetes have a gene variant (haptoglobin 2-2 gene) that increases oxidative stress and at least doubles the risk of cardiovascular disease. Israel researchers found that when these people were given vitamin E 400 IU as supplements daily, their risk of cardiovascular events such as stroke and heart attack fell by 50 percent.

- Skin health. Vitamin E has enjoyed a reputation for preventing the effects of aging on skin. As a powerful antioxidant, it is used to treat scars, acne, and wrinkles because it promotes cell regeneration of the skin. It can also reduce the sensitivity to the sun in photo-dermatitis; and when it is absorbed by the epidermis layer of the skin, it can protect against sunburn. Vitamin E oil is used on cancer patients to protect against the adverse skin effects of chemicals used in chemotherapy.

- It may have hepato-protective properties. The oxidative stress can also damage the liver, which if untreated can lead to non-alcoholic fatty liver disease (NAFLD). The best studied antioxidant for NAFLD happens to be vitamin E, with doses ranging from 400 to 1,200 IU per day. Vitamin E is found to reduce fatty infiltration of the liver.

High doses of vitamin E supplementation can be dangerous due to side effects, which can include nausea, diarrhea, stomach cramps, vomiting and heart palpitation. There is some serious concern that vitamin E might increase the chance of a hemorrhagic stroke by 22% with dosage ranges between 400—800 IU daily. Make sure you consult your physician before starting your regular vitamin E supplement, especially when you are taking medications for blood thinning (anti-platelet therapy).

Water

Though not like a vitamin or mineral, it is crucial for good health. Your body cannot survive without the supplementation of water. With age, the sense of thirst may decline; certain medications can increase your risk of becoming dehydrated, such as diuretics and stool softeners. If you are on a high-fiber diet, water is especially important because fiber absorbs water. Many of us tend to take water for granted because there is so much of it everywhere; your body is mostly water and our planet earth is also mostly water.

Ironically, a lot of people do not have sufficient levels of water in their bodies and are constantly in a state of physiological dehydration to some extent. You will not feel it right away and you usually drink only when you are thirsty. Actually you are already dehydrated at that point. Experts used to prescribe eight full glasses of water every day. The most recent advice for water consumption is that people divide their body weight in half and drink that amount of water in ounces, unless you are very active. A 160-pound person, for example, would aim for 80 ounces of water daily.

In fact, you can eat your water because many fruits and vegetables like cucumbers, lettuce, radishes and celery have water content up to 95 percent. You do not have to take in your water in liquid form in order to stay hydrated.

Instead of sugary drinks, you can add fresh fruit to your water such as a piece of lemon which will give you antioxidants and nutrients. You can replace some of your water intake with green tea.

One caution: Some of the older adults may need to have their amount of water or fluid restricted due to medical reasons such as kidney, heart or liver disease. Make sure you consult your physician about the suitable amount of fluid for you.

When you are dehydrated, regardless if it is mild or severe, it can cause health problems for your skin, muscles and mood. Your heart and kidneys and cholesterol levels will also suffer. And you will probably be eating more when you are dehydrated because your thirst can masquerade as hunger due to the fact that your brain has difficulty deciphering between thirst and hunger.

Water is involved in hundreds of biochemical reactions in your body, and let us take a look at some of the problems you may encounter when you are dehydrated, even as little as 2%:

- Dehydration leads to less efficient aerobic performance. Your heart rate goes up consuming more oxygen. This means that you will fatigue more easily and get into anaerobic metabolism that will produce lactic acid, resulting in muscle cramps and soreness. According to a study by the International Institute of Race Medicine, athletes' performance worsens even at 2 percent loss of water volume.
- Skin damage. One of the most important factors in protecting your skin is hydration; in fact, it can be the most important one. When your body is dehydrated, your skin receives less oxygen and nutrients due to decreased blood flow. The dry, rough skin is prone to wrinkles, leading to premature aging.
- A strain on your heart. Due to decreased volume, your heart has to work harder to maintain the amount of blood pumped out to various tissues and organs of your body.

- Effects on your mind and mood. When you are dehydrated, you usually don't feel well, manifesting as fatigue and exhaustion, leading to a bad mood. Even mild dehydration at 15 percent loss of normal water volume can alter a person's mood, energy level and ability to think clearly, according to two studies conducted at the University of Connecticut.

- Kidney problems. When you do not have enough water in your body, the kidneys cannot get rid of the toxins and metabolic wastes in the system. When dehydration occurs, there is a shunt of blood away from the gut and kidneys so that the blood will preferentially go to the brain and heart, a physiological protective mechanism. With decreased blood supply to the kidneys, there is less nutrients and oxygen to the kidneys, resulting in potential damage if dehydration state is not corrected in a timely fashion. The best indicator of your dehydration status is your urine. Someone who is well hydrated will produce clear to light-colored urine. Dark-colored and concentrated urine is a sign of dehydration; urine that has a strong smell can also be an indicator of dehydration.

- Swollen feet and hands. This is due to retention of salts by the kidneys, as a result of dehydration in your body.

- Headaches. Most people are not aware of this symptom from lack of enough water. Headaches caused by dehydration is fairly common in athletes. Dehydration causes the brain to shrink and pull away from the skull, eventually leading to headaches. This also lowers the oxygen supply to the brain tissues due to decreased blood flow. So, if you are running or walking or exercising and you feel the pain in your head, drink some water.

- High cholesterol levels. Dehydration during fasting increases lipid concentrations because the lack of water will make your blood thicker, elevating the levels of cholesterol correspondingly.
- Poor digestion. When your stomach does not have sufficient water to produce digestive acids or juice, this can lead to reflux and gastritis.
- Constipation. This is common among the elderly people. Water is necessary in sufficient amount for the fiber to absorb and to act as a lubricant to move the digested food and wastes down your intestinal tract.
- Bad breath. One of the functions of your saliva is anti-bacterial. If you are dehydrated, the amount of saliva produced will be diminished, which can result in a lot of bacteria growing in your oral cavity and causing bad breath, in addition to drying of your lips.

It is very important for you to stay well-hydrated, regardless of your age so that the organs of your body can function optimally.

When you get older, your nutritional needs may change. To help you make informed decision, talk to your doctor and/or dietician, in addition to your own diligence. They can work together with you to determine if your intake of a specific nutrient might be too low or too high, and then decide how you can achieve a healthy balance between the foods and nutrients you personally need.

CHAPTER EIGHT

Aging and Constipation

When I was a medical student, I had a chance to perform History and Physical Examination on many patients in nursing homes. I noticed that stool softeners and laxatives were standard routine orders on admission for the nursing home residents for any complaints of constipation. Constipation is often treated as an after-thought with very little medical attention. In fact, I ran into some nursing home residents with severe abdominal pain due to fecal compaction.

Constipation is fairly common in all age groups, but people over age 65 suffer the most. According to a recent National Institute of Health survey, over four million Americans feel constipated frequently. In general, the three factors that contribute to most of the constipation cases are: lack of exercise, a low-fiber diet, and low fluid intake. Other causes of bowel irregularity include motility problems of the gastrointestinal tract, and constipating medications such as diuretics, certain antacids, narcotics, iron supplements, calcium channel blockers, non-steroidal anti-inflammatory agents (both over-the-counter and prescriptions), antihistamine and tricyclic anti-depressants.

There is no standard rule governing the frequency of bowel movements or regularity. Most people have a bowel movement every day; some have bowel movements two to three times a day while others may have normal bowel movements every two to three days. The problem of constipation is seldom life threatening or serious, but chronic constipation can certainly disrupt a person's quality of life, and it requires medical attention to find out the causes so that it can be managed and prevented from repeatedly occurring in the future. If your symptoms of constipation persist more than two to three weeks, with bloating, abdominal pain and cramps, hard stools alternating with scanty diarrhea, your doctor should be notified and consulted in order to rule out colorectal cancer and bowel obstruction.

The older adults are at risk for constipation, especially if they have an illness and are bed-ridden for some time. Other elderly people with chronic disability and limited physical activity are also prone to having constipation. The signs and symptoms of constipation in the elderly include infrequent bowel movement or defecation, hard and lumpy stool, straining during defecation, sense of incomplete evacuation, bloating, pain in the abdomen and lack of appetite. If untreated, it can lead to complications such as fecal impaction, hemorrhoids and hemorrhoidal bleed, anal fissures and rectal prolapse. The most feared complication is bowel obstruction from persistent fecal impaction.

Some of the risk factors for constipation are already mentioned and as follows:

- Old age
- Dehydration
- Physical inactivity

- Low dietary fiber
- Depression
- Medications
- Pregnancy
- Hormonal imbalance

In general, treatments are pretty straight forward; these include diet and lifestyle changes including physical activity and regular exercise. Hydration status must be optimally maintained. Other treatments are available such as laxatives (stimulating contraction of the intestines), lubricants, stool softeners (drawing water from the intestines to the stools), and enemas (if there is fecal impaction).

There are foods that can help your bowels move and here is a list for you to incorporate them into your diet:

- Coffee. It has been shown to promote the release of gastrin, which can increase colonic motor activity.
- Chia seeds. They are a high-fiber food, and its soluble fiber becomes gelatinous when wet and helps carry away matters that might be stuck in the intestinal tract.
- Kiwi. It is a high-fiber fruit that may aid in your constipation.
- Whole milk. The extra calcium from the dairy products causes the intestines to move out more fat as opposed to it sticking around in the body.
- Probiotic yogurt. The good bacteria promotes a healthy micro-environment in the digestive tract, leading to healthy bowel movements with regularity.

- Peppermint. For people with irritable bowel syndrome, it has a calming effect on the muscles of intestinal tract, promoting regularity.
- Beans and legumes. High-fiber food that helps to bulk up your stools making it easy for them to pass through the gastrointestinal tract.
- Brown rice. Another high-fiber food good for intestinal motility. A study in 2007 found that women who consumed brown rice lowered their chances of getting constipation by 47 percent than those who did not eat brown rice.
- Bananas. Another high-fiber fruit that promote bowel motility. With their insoluble fiber, bananas can help you push out digestive wastes better by making stools easier to transit through. They also contain some probiotics that are crucial for healthy microbes in the guts.
- Prunes. They are dried plums with high fiber content, and are great for keeping your bowel movements regular.
- Avocados. They have high magnesium content which helps keep moisture in the guts, thus softening the stools and increasing the flow.
- Pears. They have some fiber, but not as much as other fruits. However, they have sorbitol, which is a sugar alcohol acting like a laxative to help increase bowel movements.
- Apples. Like pears, their skin contains most of the insoluble fiber that helps to move things along in your intestinal tract.
- Peaches. Besides fiber, they also have a high content of sorbitol which promotes bowel movements.
- Cashew nuts. They are a good source of magnesium, which is essential for a healthy passage of stools.

- Plain popcorn. They are high in fiber and low in calories. The more fiber you take in, the more bulk it adds to your stools, making it easier to get down the gastrointestinal tract for elimination. Forget about the popcorn you get at the cinema.
- Broccoli and cauliflowers. Rich in fiber content besides their other important nutrients.
- Blackberries and raspberries. These little things carry more fiber than other berries and are loaded with healthy antioxidants.
- Oatmeal. A bowl of oatmeal in the morning is a good way to get your digestive tract moving due to its high fiber content.
- Plums. They are a great source of sorbitol and fiber, ideal for bowel movement.
- Water. Last but not least, make sure you keep up with your needs for water to stay well-hydrated. All the intake of fiber from food requires water to work efficiently.

Note: Fiber is also known as roughage, and it is the indigestible portion of healthy, unprocessed foods. It comes in two forms: insoluble and soluble. Insoluble fiber adds bulk to your stool and thus alleviates constipation, while soluble fiber forms a gel when wet in your digestive system to increase feelings of fullness and can help reduce cholesterol levels. For your information, fiber is not found in animal products.

CHAPTER NINE

Aging and Frailty

Frailty is something that most people who live to an advanced age will face. Incidence of frailty increase with age from 3.9 percent in 65—74 age group to 25 percent in the 85+ group. The incidence of occurrence is higher in women than men. African Americans were more than twice as likely to be frail than Caucasians (13% versus 6% according to the studies). It is becoming a worldwide problem and challenge, facing countries with aging populations.

A recent survey of 7,510 community-dwelling older adults in 10 European countries found that prevalence of frailty ranged from 5.8% in Switzerland to 27% in Spain, according to some studies. Community-dwelling means NOT living in nursing homes or hospitals.

Frailty is a geriatric syndrome in the elderly population, characterized by diffuse weakness, weight loss and very limited physical activity that is associated with adverse health outcomes. Frailty typically manifests itself as an age-related biological vulnerability to stressors and decreased physiological reserves, leading to a limited capacity to maintain homeostasis.

There are five widely recognized and accepted criteria to characterize the geriatric syndrome of frailty, established by Dr. Linda Fried:

- Weakness by the decrease in grip strength
- Unintentional weight loss, ten pounds or more in the past year
- Self-reported exhaustion
- Slow walking speed
- Low physical activity

Here are the characteristic descriptive features: shrinking, weakening, slowing, weight-losing and energy-lacking.

Frail people usually suffer from three or more of the five criteria. Frailty, undoubtedly, is going to be more common because people are living longer, both in the developed and developing countries. It can affect how elderly persons will respond to medical treatment, as well as how long and how well they will live. Most people will not have difficulty recognizing frailty, they will know it when they see it. However, the phenomenon of frailty remains poorly understood at this time despite on-going investigation and research. In general, it has been shown that patients who are frail have poorer outcomes when faced with any stress like surgery or a new major illness.

Frailty, nowadays, is considered a medical condition, not an inevitable part of aging because most of the older adults are not frail and they will never get frail. Many medical experts believe that frailty can be prevented or delayed, and can even be reversed in older people with regular screening to assess their vulnerability to developing frailty so that appropriate interventions can be implemented in a timely manner.

Our nation's increasing longevity is bringing new challenges for health and social programs. American life span in 2009 was 78.5 years, according to the data provided by the Center for Disease Control and Prevention, about three decades more life than 1900, when the life expectancy was 47.3 years. We have added 30 years to the human life span in the U.S., which is a proud success for public health, medicine, and education.

With the rapid rate of growth in the population 65 and older, the number of frail elderly people is definitely increasing every year. The frail older adults present special challenges for all of us in the society; they need to involve physicians specialized in geriatric medicine, social workers, care-takers, physical and occupational therapists, nutritionist/dieticians, psychologists/councilors, spiritual leaders or chaplains and family members who are looking after the frail parents. They are weak, often have multiple medical problems, limited ability for independent living, may have impaired mental function, and often require assistance for daily activities such as eating, dressing and toileting.

Researchers have found some parameters that can be strongly linked to Frailty Syndrome. Most specifically, the plasma levels of the inflammatory marker, IL-6, are elevated in the frail people. Among the lipid parameters, the decreases of total cholesterol and HDL-C were found to be very strongly associated with Frailty Syndrome. The weak to moderate associations were found in the nutritional and coagulation parameter.

According to researchers at Johns Hopkins University School of Medicine, they believe that frailty may in part be related to the body's inability to regulate normal inflammatory responses. Dr. Jeremy D. Watson, a geriatrician and molecular biologist at the Biology of Healthy Aging Program at Johns Hopkins University has found that frail people suffer from a constant low-grade inflammatory state. Frail people, as observed, are less able to metabolize glucose properly, and secrete more cortisol, a stress hormone, which over time increases chronic inflammation and damage the skeletal muscles and immune system.

Hormonal changes with age have been suspected of causing some of the problems seen in frailty. Both estrogen in women and testosterone in men when decreased with age can lead to the decline in muscle mass. Also elevated cortisol and reduced vitamin D levels may contribute to frailty according to research studies.

The physiological characteristics of frailty such as poor muscle strength, exhaustion, limited physical activity and unintentional weight loss can be partially explained by the increased levels of inflammatory markers, especially, IL-6. This cytokine, together with C-Reactive Protein, is one of the most studied parameters which are strongly associated with the Frailty Syndrome.

HDL is a powerful anti-inflammatory agent, a decrease of which is related to an increase of inflammatory state. Lipids play important roles in cellular metabolisms and the cell membranes; their abnormal levels would cause altered cellular function in all organs. This chronic inflammatory state can lead to sarcopenia, prevalent in the elderly, healthy or not. IL-6 is an important factor modulating muscle mass and strength and ultimately causing sarcopenia and reduction in bone density.

Inflammation should be considered an important target for prevention and intervention in the care of the frail elderly population. Despite some reservations, it is still worthwhile to try to intervene.

Other preventive and interventional measures for the frail elderly group should include:

- Nutritional support, with proteins in particular. I think the frail elderly people should receive all the necessary vitamins and minerals, and some may need the levels greater than the recommended daily values due to their limited physiological reserves, as long as any toxicity and side effects are being watched.
- Supplementation with sex hormones and growth hormone is a potential intervention to improve muscle mass and strength. However, due to potential serious side effects, no hormonal therapy is recommended for frail older adults at this time.
- Physical therapy for resistance exercise, strength and balance. Poor balance is a common cause of falls among seniors, resulting in broker hips and head injuries. One in three people aged 65 and older will suffer a fall. Gait-training is very important so that frail patients can resume regular walking.

   The focus of balance training is on the ability of the joints and brain to communicate. The balance system is in the ears (the vestibular system), and vision. Improved balance will improve confidence and level of mobility.

   Resistance exercises, structured according to the older adults abilities, are useful to build muscles and help to reduce joint stiffness and pain. Even a small increase in physical fitness can improve symptoms of frailty.
- Vision check. As you get older, your vision changes because your lenses in the eyes tend to lose their flexibility to focus. All frail older adults should have a comprehensive dilated eye examination annually. If you can't see where you are going,

your fall risk goes up. Cataracts and glaucoma can occur at any age, but most often they happen to people over 60. Age-related macular degeneration (AMD) is common in the older adults, and can cause blindness.

- Diet with fruits and vegetables which are rich in antioxidants to decrease inflammation, improve blood flow, and boost the immune system. Fiber helps to decrease cholesterol and regulate blood sugar. The healthy diet should also include lutein, omega-3 fatty acids, vitamin C and E to promote eye health. Food should be tasty and easy to swallow and digest, and to prevent malnutrition and under-nutrition.

- Recognize and treat depression. Depression is a major cause of anorexia and weight loss in the elder people. With so many adverse events going on in the bodies of the frail older adults, there has to be deep seated depression, which, as can be expected, leads to slowing of the physical activity and thought processes. Depressed people are more likely to develop major illnesses such as myocardial infarction and stroke.

- Keep their mind active. Crossword puzzles, reading, playing games, watching comedies, and socializing are excellent ways to maintain mental sharpness and slow cognitive decline.

- Safety. We must pay attention to several aspects of safety within the frail community. First and foremost, it is the personal safety of the residents/patients. Visitors including friends and relatives should be screened so that nobody can take advantage of them. Structural safety within the premises probably will go beyond the standard building codes with some variations due to the unique medical conditions of the frail people. Safeguards should be in place when the frail older adults socializing outdoors or going on a field trip.

Depression and despair can be sadly assumed to be found in all of the frail older adults; they are experiencing loss of any notion of invincibility, loss of the ability to take care of themselves in their daily life, and loss of possibility of a subsequent life stage. All age survivors on average deteriorate from agility in their 60s—80s to a period of frailty preceding death. This deterioration is gradual for some and precipitous for others.

The scary thing about getting older is the thought of losing your independence. It is a sad fact that by age 70, 25% of your muscle mass is gone which contribute to the loss of independence. Majority of people who broke their hips seldom fully regain their independence.

But, there is no reason to give up or give in to the symptoms of aging. There is a lot you can do to improve your chances of staying active and living independently in your own home for your whole life. Statistically, one third of older adults over age 65 have mobility problems. Many of them will end up having to move from their homes.so they get the care they need. But, it doesn't have to be this way!

Frail older adults require a high level of care. Medical advances have made it possible to ' postpone death ' for years. This added time costs many frail people prolonged sickness, dependence, pain and suffering. These final years are, no doubt, costly in economic terms. According to Medicare reports, one out of every four dollars is spent on the frail in the last year of life, in attempts to postpone death. Some experts in Medical Ethics suggest that medical treatments in the final days are not only economically costly, they are often unnecessary. I personally disagree.

The frail older adults comprise one particularly vulnerable population, which has drawn some controversy. I am going to mention a couple of organizations that are trying to deal with the situations.

Aging With Dignity. This is a national non-profit organization based in Tallahassee, Florida. Its primary focus is to improve end-of-life care by encouraging people to make medical decisions in advance of a serious illness. Its stated mission is to ' honor the God-given human dignity of the most vulnerable among us '.

They developed Five Wishes for anyone 18 or older and is used in all 50 states and in many countries. It meets the legal requirements for an advance directive in at least 42 states of the U.S. and the District of Columbia. In the other states, your completed Five Wishes can be attached to your state's requited for.

Dignity In Dying. It is an organization in the United Kingdom (UK). Their stated primary aim is campaigning for individuals to have greater choice and more control over end-of-life decisions, so as to alleviate any suffering they may be undergoing as they near the end of their life. They include providing terminally ill adults with the option of a painless, assisted death within strict legal safeguards. The organization declares that its campaign looks to bring about a generally more compassionate approach to the end-of-life.

Caring for the frail older adults is very challenging and intensive, medically complex, with increased social needs. Efforts of intervention should be focusing on the prevention of functional decline and improvement of functional independence. I personally propose and support the concept of Frailty Compassionate Care Center (FCCC), which will decrease the frequency of hospitalization, and emergency room visits, which often provide superficial care for the frail older patients without results of functional improvements or quality of life.

The FCCC should be a community for the frail elderly, unlike nursing homes and private homes. The setting should be a safe place, both internally and externally. The caring team should consist of a physician specialized in geriatric medicine, psychologists and counselors, nurses, physical and occupational therapists, social workers, chaplains for their spiritual needs, trained care takers (assistants), and family members. The residents in the Center receive complete long term care and are followed until the end of their lives.

In fact, many retirement centers can establish a Frailty Care Unit on premise, just like Alzheimer's Unit some already have.

The FCCC should be a joint effort, or establishment by the Government, faith organizations, volunteers, and benefactors from private enterprises; it should be protected from any frivolous legal liabilities. We must realize and understand that our Government cannot do it alone and should not be expected to provide everything from cradle to grave, especially for the frail elderly population which is getting larger and larger, and it might include you in the future if you live long enough and become frail. After all, we know that about 25 percent of the older adults in their 80s will face the reality of frailty, either happening to you gradually or precipitously.

CHAPTER TEN

Aging and Walking

Nobody can deny the health benefits of exercise, but when you are aging past 65 or older, realistically and actually, there are only a few forms of age-appropriate exercise that are safe and practicable and easy to start for the elderly population. The one that stands out as the most important and convenient is walking. Walking is the exercise you can enjoy and benefit from even at ripe old age without causing damage to your joints. Walking is a low-impact exercise and can be done for longer periods of time; it can also help you reach your fitness and weight-loss goals. At this stage, you are looking for mobility, stability and balance, NOT intense huge gain or speed. Many studies have shown that regular, daily walking is integral to your health and longevity.

However, there are many factors that can play into having a long, healthy life including heredity, diet and the social determinants of health such as where you live (environmental), and your economic stability. But, one determinant which is often-underestimated and sometimes neglected is your mobility; it is your ability to move freely and without or tolerable pain. In fact, many studies have shown that mobility can predict the quality of life, especially in older adults, since limited mobility is associated with poorer physical and mental health outcomes, limited access to healthcare services and increased risk of falls and other injuries.

The vast, almost innumerable health benefits of walking as an exercise on cardiovascular, physical and mental health are incontrovertible. Physical inactivity is the culprit of the disease process for many chronic, degenerative states. The most important and necessary thing for human survival, after oxygen, water, salt and food, is movement which includes walking. Human beings are meant to walk; we are bipedal, erect species with bodies designed for locomotion.

Age is a risk factor for the development of Alzheimer's disease, which accounts for about 70% of all dementia cases. In the early stages of this neurodegenerative illness, the affected individuals are generally ambulatory, able to use and move their arms and legs freely, unless they are also suffering from debilitating co-morbidities. The patients have a " golden window of opportunity " to improve and maintain their physical and mental well-being while their muscle memories are essentially intact.

Walking is a complex behavior and a very important, bodily function. Walking requires functional integration of a lot of sensory and motor interaction and experience; it activates the brain and the musculoskeletal system. One of the important components of walking is balancing. In order to maintain the body's balance unconsciously and effortlessly as it changes position and moves over somewhat uneven terrain in a gravitational field, the brain needs and interacts with different information. It relies partly on a mechanism in the inner ears responsible for sensory orientation in three-dimensional space. If this function of inner ears fails, you cannot maintain equilibrium or balance.

Besides the ears, the brain also requires visual input of information from other senses to keep the walking person in balance: from the tactile receptors which let the brain know which part of the body is in contact with the ground, and from the proprioceptors in the muscles, tendons and joints that keep the brain continuously informed of the exact position of each part of the body in space. Dysfunction in any of these neuronal circuitries can lead to erratic movements and falling.

The cerebellum, located below the occipital lobes of the cerebrum, processes all of these sensory input to coordinate responses of muscles to the ever-changing requirements of ambulation. Research shows that exercise stimulates the sensory and motor cortex and maintains the brain's balance system. These functions begin to deteriorate gradually as we get older, making us prone to falling and becoming home-bound and bed-confined. Nothing accelerates atrophy of the brain more than being immobilized in the same environment with little stimulation.

Normal walking involves movements of the limbs in cross-patterned fashion; the right leg and the left arm move forward at the same time, then the left leg and the right arm. Researchers believe that the cross-patterned movements seem to have a harmonizing influence on the Central Nervous System while generating electrical activities in the brain, and bolster normal development and optimal functioning of the human brain.

Researchers of observational studies believe that when the babies first start to crawl, their cross-patterned movements serve to stimulate optimal brain development. This coordinated movements of crawling may look regressive and odd for the grown-ups, especially for those who have difficulty walking, but it may be a good exercise for the brain. Some older adults may want to try crawling on a clean carpeted floor with the caregivers around, and have some good workout. Personally, I think there is nothing to lose in terms of physical and mental health, and everything to gain!

An eye-opening experiment was conducted by Swedish psychologist, Dr. Bengt Saltin, who had five volunteers for three weeks to assist him in the study of extended bed-rest on the body. The five young men in the experiment were physically fit, but at the end of the three weeks laying in beds, all of them showed a reduction in the aerobic capacity that equated with twenty years of aging. The experiment confirmed the paramount importance of bodily movements and exercise in maintaining and promoting good health and slowing the aging process.

Let us look at the numerous science-backed health benefits from regular walking 25 to 30 minutes a day, at least five days a week:

- Walking for stronger bones—As we age, we lose the ability to absorb sufficient calcium into the body and the bones become thinner, leading to osteoporosis. Osteoporosis is a common cause of fractures among the elderly, hip fractures in particular. Statistically, hip fractures strike at least one out of three women and one out of six men. Walking stimulates the body's assimilation of calcium and other nutrients.

  A gradual exposure to the sunlight when walking could be a wonderful and natural way to increase calcium absorption into the body and bones to minimize and/or prevent osteoporosis. Studies have shown that walking increases bone mass (bone density), not only in the legs, but also the arms. It is so important to be vigilant and cautious to avoid accidental falls or any injury that can result in fractures, which will set you back with immobilization, potentially subjecting you to many health problems.

- Walking can help lowering the blood pressure—the walking movements open up the capillaries in the muscle tissues by reducing the resistance to blood flow in the arterial beds, causing the blood pressure to drop. That's why walking is recommended for people with hypertension among other things. Many researchers have shown and agreed that a normal blood pressure helps to lower the risk of cardiovascular disease, stroke and Alzheimer's disease.

- Walking can help decrease swelling in the lower extremities— the contraction and relaxation of the leg muscles during walking help mobilize and overcome the force of gravity. Thus, the blood pooling in the leg veins (the venous system) is pushed upward (proximally) against gravity by frequent contractions of muscles in the lower extremities.

  This also causes an equally effective flow within the lymphatic system and decrease edema in the legs; in other words, walking can help eliminate swelling in both the venous and lymphatic systems.

- Walking burns glucose and decreases insulin resistance— As one gets older, insulin sensitivity decreases; studies have demonstrated that walking can improve insulin sensitivity and lower blood glucose levels. In other words, walking can help management of diabetes; a well-controlled diabetic means lower risk for diseases such as cardiovascular and Alzheimer's.

- Walking, like other aerobic exercises, stimulates the release of endorphins in the brain and help fight stress and depression, improving your mood and sleep.

- Walking clearly improves circulation and the elasticity of the arteries, according to many studies, making the heart a more efficient pump, thus enhancing cerebral circulation and providing more oxygen and nutrients to the brain. Optimal cerebral blood flow undoubtedly can decrease the risk for the development of Alzheimer's disease and stroke, making you feel mentally sharper.

- Walking promotes the movements of the intestines, bolstering and enhancing peristalsis, thereby helping constipation, which is a common problem for the geriatric group. It is physiologically crucial to have efficient elimination of metabolic wastes to maintain optimal functions of the body including the brain, achieving homeostasis.

- Walking can help lose weight—walking, often taken for granted with its beneficent nature neglected and/or under-valued, is a good form of exercise to help you reach your fitness and weight-loss goals. It is time to change that attitude and misconception. Many studies have shown that not only can you lose weight by doing it, but the more you weigh, the easier it is for you to realize the pounds being dropped. Nevertheless, it varies from person to person as to how much weight and how fast you can lose by walking routine. You must remind yourself that good health is a long-term goal and cannot be achieved quickly.

There is no magic formula for how many steps, miles, or hours you must walk to lose the amount of weight that you want. If you have a sedentary desk job, a walk every evening after dinner may surprise you with real results. There are many talks about a baseline of 10,000 steps a day; if you are able to do more, you will realize better bodily functions and feel better.

If you can, try to challenge yourself with intervals—periods of faster walking. Research has found that interval walkers lose more weight than people who just go the same speed all the time. So, you will get more bang for your buck by increasing your walking pace at intervals.

- Walking is known to decrease the amount of undesirable body fats and the levels of serum cholesterol with less deposits within the arterial walls, thus, reducing the occurrence of atherosclerosis. We know that atherosclerosis, indisputably, is a major risk for heart attack and stroke, and stroke is a significant contributing factor for up to 30% of Alzheimer's cases, according to the findings at autopsies of Alzheimer's patients.

- Walking can help tone the respiratory system and increase the exchanges of oxygen and carbon dioxide. By age 65, the lungs lose as much as 40% of their capacity to utilize oxygen, this is partly due to the decreasing numbers of alveoli and corresponding capillaries of the lungs with aging.

- Walking and other exercise can help lower the levels of oxidative stress, according to many research studies. Reduced levels of oxidative stress in the body are associated with reduced formation of beta-amyloid plaques, one of the two pathophysiological features of Alzheimer's disease. However, vigorous and intense exercises often cause considerable oxidative stress due to higher demand for energy, and it is difficult to know at what point you begin to do more harm than good. It is generally accepted that it is more beneficial with more gentle/mild aerobic exercise, like walking and leisurely swimming.

- Walking can increase the release of brain derived neurotrophic factor (BDNF), a protective protein in the brain, and this is found to improve learning and memory, according to many neuroscientific studies. In a 2011 meta-analysis of 15 studies that followed more than 33,000 people for up to 12 years, physical activity including walking provided a buffer against cognitive decline and poor memory with its many other health benefits, both physically and mentally.

According to neuroscientific research, exercise stimulates the production and release of BDNF, a neuronal growth factor, which plays a crucial role in effecting neuroplasticity and cognitive function. Simply walking at a good pace has been shown to bolster the growth of new neurons; patients with Alzheimer's disease tend to have reduced BDNF levels compared to healthy, normal individuals.

- Walking, like other forms of exercise, is a powerful stimulator of ' mitochondrial biogenesis '. Studies have shown that aerobic exercise can increase the number and size of mitochondria in muscles, allowing the muscles to become more efficient at extracting oxygen from the blood. Research further has demonstrated that energy shortage in the brain due to dysfunctional mitochondria can increase the levels of the precursor for formation of the beta-amyloid plaques.

- Walking can slow down the progress of age-related changes of the brain, i.e. tissue loss or decrease in the cerebral cortex, hippocampus and the cerebral white matter. If unchecked, the amount of tissue shrinkage from the aging process is most dramatic in the hippocampus, as much as 30% according to some research.

The nerve conduction time also decreases with age due to demyelination. Research has shown that physical activity and aerobic exercise can retard such age-related changes and facilitate re-innervation of damaged nerves.

- When walking, it is good and healthy to look at distant objects because looking at the distance helps to relax the ciliary muscles and suspensory ligaments of the lens of the eyes. This can help to decrease the risk of age-related macular degeneration, which is a common cause of blindness among the elderly people.

  When you are walking, enjoy the fresh air and nature, connecting with the nature spiritually. Walking outdoors allows you to decompress and refocus. Many studies have shown that our spiritual connections improve the immune system and depressive moods. Many studies have shown that walking is nature's effective and inexpensive anti-depressant, especially for someone with Alzheimer's disease and still capable of walking.

Movement is a natural function, and it should be maintained, if at all possible and as long as possible. Walking can help increase a sense of well-being and vitality; it can also improve physical and mental health for anyone, and the older generation needs it even more. There are two ways we can maintain the overall, optimal function of our brain: one is by creating new neurons, and the other is by extending the life of existing neurons. Physical activity and learning something new essentially work in complementary fashion: physical activity can help make new neurons and new learning can help prolong neurons' survival.

Our bodies are made for movements, whether you walk slowly or rapidly, it makes little difference in terms of health benefits. In fact, if you can take a walk after a meal or dinner, you will have better digestion, you will have less gas with better peristalsis, you will stabilize your blood sugar levels better, and you will feel generally better with less stress.

A few words of caution for the elderly:

- Never attempt to walk alone
- Make sure that the terrain is relatively level and without visual obstruction
- Try to look for and pick a visual target
- Be familiar with the walking area so that you will not become a victim of crime
- Take some rest at intervals if needed, especially you are in the beginning of this worthwhile endeavor
- Avoid noisy and crowded surroundings to minimize distraction

CHAPTER ELEVEN

Spirituality and Faith

Spirituality is personal and private, it is self-enhancing, it is connecting, and it is peace-loving. Spirituality is part of being human. Just as all of us have a physical aspect, and an emotional aspect, we also have a spiritual aspect. You are mistaken if you assume that you do not have a spiritual aspect if you do not believe in God. You may discover some very surprising and moving spiritual focuses and effects in your life if you have the courage to explore this part of your makeup.

Spirituality is an inviting word when it is understood. It invites you to discover your world of values and beliefs. In other words, aging is a spiritual journey and spirituality is the essential piece of every person's aging process.

Many scientists who studied spirituality and aging have concluded that spirituality increases with age. In the past few decades, gerontologists have become increasingly aware of the importance of spirituality to the well-being of the elderly people.

The word ' spirit ' is derived from the Latin spiritus, meaning ' soul, courage, vigor, breath '. Thus, the spirit is our vital center or our core. Spiritual experiences are those events in life and moments in relationships which attune us to that vital force within and which give us meaning and depth in our day-to-day living. The process of aging in every life stage can bring about changes in your spiritual life.

Spirituality can include religious faith and practices, but can also be experienced and understood in non-religious ways. Spirituality is not the same as religion!

Aging and spirituality are interwoven in a mystical and awe-inspiring way. Spirituality provides shelter for the aging and at the same time it makes the aging process a wonderful journey. In the confines of spirituality, the fear of aging will disappear. The cells of your body will benefit and you will have a greater sense of wellness. Studies have shown that spirituality strengthens the mind. When your mind becomes strong, your body will follow suit.

Fear and anxiety are powerful negative forces, which are common in the elderly people. Spirituality can and will provide you with the foundation to minimize the effect of fear and anxiety and help you reconcile with your sense of self. Fear of dying is often associated with the aging older adults, and spirituality can help you subdue that fear.

Practicing spirituality can help you remain positive in life and face illnesses with more strength. As you get older, your body will go through many changes. Your immune system is becoming weaker and less efficient, making you prone to illnesses. Along with a weakening mind, the body will have difficulty recovering from illnesses.

Several philosophical teachers and spiritual leaders, from Plato to Eckhart Tolle, had written books that highlight aging and spirituality. But at the core of it lies the fact that spirituality will help you re-define the sense of purpose. The point of bringing a spiritual perspective into your life is to remind yourself that you are more than just your own physical own body, and that there is more to life than the material world. We are actually spiritual beings inhabiting the material/physical forms. I believe, nothing is random in life: the miraculous make-up of the human body, the wonders of nature, the complex and inexplicable creation of birth, and the profound earthly journey from the beginning to the end.

What is spiritual healing?

The term refers to healing transmitted by the spirit or divine force through faith, in the presence of a healer. Sometimes, the healer may not be physically present as long as there is an awareness. The concept of spiritual healing is found in all cultures and societies. In Europe, North America, South America, Asia and Africa, people versed in the care of the divine soul or spirit have sought and tried to cure those who have become sick.

Spiritual care involves the whole person—the physical, emotional, social, and spiritual. In delivering this care, physicians need to understand the spiritual dimensions in patients' lives and may have to talk about what is important to them.

Spirituality seems to be receiving more and more attention in the medical community, with national recognition of the value of spiritual care. The Joint Commission on Accreditation of Healthcare Organization has a policy that states: " For many patients, pastoral care and other spiritual services are an integral part of health care and daily life. The hospital is able to provide pastoral care and other spiritual services for patients who request them ".

In 1992, three medical schools offered courses on spirituality and health. In 2001, 75 medical schools offered such courses and many of these courses are required. At the George Washington University School of Medicine, spirituality is interwoven with the rest of the curriculum throughout the four years of medical school training so that all medical students learn to integrate it into all of patients care. Since the goal of good medical care is attention to the whole person, not just the specific disease or illness. Furthermore, one of the basic premises of these special courses is that focusing on the spiritual aspect of patients enables physicians to deliver more compassionate care. It has become clear that medical school faculty find the topic of spirituality and health relevant to medical education and patient care.

Dr. Victor Frankl, a psychiatrist who described his experiences in a Nazi concentration camp, wrote: " Man is not destroyed by suffering; he is destroyed by suffering without meaning ". One of the challenges physicians face is to help the aging people find meaning and acceptance in the midst of pain and suffering and chronic illness. Medical ethicists of our time have reminded us that religion and spirituality form the basis of meaning and purpose for many people. Healing can be experienced as acceptance of illness and peace with one's life, and this healing is at its core spiritual!

The effect of spirituality on health is an area of active research right now, by physicians, psychologists and other professionals. The focus of their studies are on three areas: mortality, coping and recovery.

Mortality

Many studies have shown that people who are spiritual tend to live longer. One research study of 1,700 older adults found that those who attended church had lower levels of the inflammatory marker, IL-6, than the non-church goers. The researcher hypothesized that religious commitments might improve stress control due to better coping mechanism, available social support and networking and the strength of personal values.

Coping

Some studies conclude that spiritual people tend to have more positive outlook and a better quality of life. Despite their illness and suffering, they feel less pain and are happier, and are satisfied with their meaningful personal existence.

The American Pain Society distributed a pain questionnaire to hospitalized patients with major painful illnesses and found that personal prayer was the most commonly used non-drug method for controlling pain. In this study, prayer as a method of pain management was used more frequently than intravenous pain medications, intra-muscular pain injections and therapeutic massages.

According to a study from the University of Florida in Gainesville and Wayne State University in Detroit, Michigan, older adults use prayer more than other alternative therapy for health; 96% of the study participants use prayers, specifically to cope with stress.

Spiritual beliefs can help patients cope with diseases and face death. A random Gallup poll asked people what concerns they would have if they were dying. Their top concerns were finding companionship and spiritual comfort—chosen over such things as advance directives, economic and financial issues, and social concerns. The most comforting spiritual reassurance is that they will be in the loving presence of God or a higher power, and that death is not the end but a passage.

Other studies found that when people are challenged by a serious illness or loss of a loved one, they frequently turn to spiritual recourses to help them cope with or understand their illness or loss.

Recovery

A study of heart transplant patients showed that those who participated in religious activities and said their beliefs were important complied better with follow-up treatment, had improved physical functioning, had higher levels of self-esteem, and had less anxiety and fewer health worries. Spirituality can certainly enhance recovery from illness and surgery due to the power of hope and positive thinking. Many other studies have also shown that spiritual practices can improve health outcomes.

Spirituality and health are inextricably and profoundly linked as more and more studies have found, and this is observed in many different cultures of the world. Metaphysically, life lives at the expense of other life. It does not matter whether you are a carnivore, omnivore or a vegetarian, you sustain and perpetuate your physical existence by taking the lives of other organisms.

Life is indeed full of changes and vicissitudes; the longer you live, the more changes you will encounter. Changes can be uplifting, challenging and energizing; sometimes they can be disheartening and devastating such as the diagnosis of Alzheimer's disease or incurable cancer, enough to shake you to your roots. What sustains and bolsters you, and keeps you steady and resilient when it feels as though the earth is shaking and moving beneath your feet? For many people, the answer is their faith. Faith means not only a belief in a Higher Power, but also social connections to others.

Many people today tend to under-value and doubt faith, assuming that it means believing without any real proof or evidence. Faith to me is more than belief; it is not gullibility, and it is not superstition. We must keep an open mind; there is a saying that " absence of evidence is NOT evidence of absence ". Faith is very personal, close to you and deep within you. Faith focuses on something hoped for, but has not yet happened. Faith is imbued with gratitude for something positive experienced, which is observable, but not measurable like in a laboratory. In essence, our physical eyes cannot see the realities in the spiritual realm.

When you have faith, you know that you are never alone in your struggle. Faith is ineffable, and to some, mysterious. The faithfuls do not need science to support their convictions because they don't require them. There is a lot of overlapping with spirituality and faith (religion), and the health benefits for the body and mind are essentially the same or very similar.

Psychoneuroimmunology, a field of medical science that studies how your mind influences your health and how social and psychological factors, such as religion, affect the immune and nervous systems. The impact of faith in the lives of almost 80% of the world's population who are involved in organized religion is enormous and undeniable. There is a growing body of evidence in social and psychological science studies that religious people are happier, healthier, and recovering better after traumas than non-religious people. Comparing with the non-religious and non-spiritual individuals, people active in their religion report greater social support, most likely, through the church or other organizational establishment itself, and live longer and recover sooner and better from illnesses.

The power of praying, either for yourself or another person, is inexplicable but observable. In our world of modern science, it is controversial because it is difficult to measure or quantify the impact of one's prayers. However, many studies have shown that praying for oneself and intercessory prayers can actually lead to positive results.

In summary, I pray that spirituality will continue to gain recognition in our social fabrics, because it is an important element in the way many of us, if not all, face chronic illness, suffering, and loss in aging.

CHAPTER TWELVE

Epilogue and Happy Aging

Some religion, like Buddhism, simply put, is the pursuit of true happiness.

According to studies done in 2012, Denmark was at the top in life satisfaction and work-life balance, and seventeenth in income. By comparison, the United States ranks No. 1 in income but 12th in life-work satisfaction and 29th in work-life balance. There is no evidence to show that money buys happiness.

Getting older has its perks; for one, you are good at what you have learned and it is called ' crystalized intelligence '. This will keep getting better, even when you are 70 and older.

In terms of happiness, a boost in your mood is linked to the release of serotonin, endorphins and oxytocin, your feel-good hormones and chemicals in your brain. Tryptophan, an amino acid, helps your body make serotonin, and so it is linked to feeling good, too. Dopamine is also a feel-good chemical that is involved in pleasure. A study found that when people listened to music, especially their favorite ones, their brains released more dopamine.

By the way, happiness is not the absence of sadness. When you suppress sadness, you are suppressing other, more positive emotions as well. People who try to suppress sadness and other emotions actually become more anxious and depressed.

In a recent survey of more than 340,000 people, age 55 and older, the researchers found that the overall feelings of well-being improve as people pass middle age. They suggest that the older adults seem to worry less than the younger ones in general because with age comes increased wisdom and emotional intelligence. They further suggest that older people might control their emotions better, and focus more on how to make the most of life.

Happiness is not a rare phenomenon; it is everywhere for you to find. Let us look at some of the ways and means that can help elevate your mood to be happy.

- Count your blessings. When you make an effort to look on the bright side, it helps you stay focused on the positives. Getting older can come with many ' thank you '; grateful for grandchildren, good health you are enjoying, more free time, wearing what you want, chance to travel and see the world, and being able to give back to the community. Gratitude brings you happiness.
- Listen to your favorite music. Music can have a powerful effect on your emotions and mood. Besides, it helps to fill the void and promote the release of feel-good chemicals in the brain.
- Practice meditation. No special equipment or physical ability is required. Meditating for even one hour a week will give you a dose of joy, peace and contentment. It will also create new

pathways in your brain to make it easier for you to feel joy. Interestingly, the Dalai Lama from Tibet, China, has become a key reference point for meditation research in the past several years. Studies have shown that meditation can reduce stress, lower blood pressure, decrease pain and enhance health.

- Cognitive re-structuring, or reframing. Aging has its share of adversity, losses, and sorrows. What makes the big difference is your attitude about them. For example, if your bad knees stop you from jogging, you do not have to despair; you can take up swimming. So, try to focus on the positive aspects of the present, not the regrets of the past or the worries about the future. You will find yourself a much happier person by doing that.

- Be generous. It is scientifically proven that giving back and helping others makes us happier and more content. Giving is a universal spiritual value taught by every religion, and the desire to give back naturally increases as we age. Generosity is truly a spiritual practice.

- Be curious and make connections. Find new friends and open to new relationships, while maintaining your life-long connections. Studies show that the more connected you are, the happier you are. It is important to cultivate your curiosity as you age. Physical exercise helps grow new muscles, mental activities help grow new brain cells, and emotional engagement lifts the spirit. Children are naturally curious, and you can be too.

Humans are social creatures by our very nature. Many psychosocial studies have shown that social connections including interactions with family and friends reduce the risk of death from coronary heart disease, strokes and chronic illnesses such as Alzheimer's disease. In the U.S., at least one in ten Americans live alone, and many are at risk for loneliness. Most of these lonely individuals are older, and the trend will continue because the geriatric population is the fastest growing segment of the world. Loneliness is " a disease of disconnection " which keeps you emotionally and socially isolated.

Psychosocial researches have further shown that lonely people experience more insomnia, more depression, more susceptible to infections due to suppressed or less effective immune system. Lonely people face greater risk of premature death from all illnesses. People who have mutually caring interpersonal relationships enjoy increased sense of well-being and mental health, display greater emotional resilience, and live longer and happier lives.

In a recent international study published in the Journal of the American Geriatric Society, it further illustrates just how detrimental loneliness can be to one's health and longevity, and it is especially bad for people who are over 60. Loneliness has significant impacts on one's quality of life. As of 2020, the numbers of adults aged over 30 made up half the total global population, marking the beginning of an increasingly aging world. As a consequence, loneliness among seniors has become an important issue of social and public health concern.

- Volunteering. Try to find ways to get involved in your community or help out someone in need. It will improve your mental health and well-being and give you peace and happiness. Just research the many opportunities of volunteering, which can come in different form, shape and settings to fit you in.

- Let it go and forgive. Are you still holding a grudge? Let it go. Forgiveness will free you from negative thoughts and bitterness, and make more room in your life for inner peace, leading to happiness. Hostility increases the risk of heart disease, according to studies by the Department of Behavioral Medicine at Duke University Medical Center. People who are hostile and bitter are more likely to have higher cholesterol and blood pressure and develop irregular heart rhythm. All of these problems can be due heightened levels of stress hormone, cortisol, and increased inflammation in the walls of coronary arteries.

When our inner world is disrupted, it is difficult to concentrate on anything other than our internal turmoil or pain. Forgiveness is about goodness, about extending mercy to ourselves and to those who have harmed us. It is not easy, but it is well worth it. Working on forgiveness can help us increase our self-esteem and give us a sense of inner strength, equanimity and safety. Many studies have shown that forgiving others can promotes strong psychological benefits such as decreasing depression, anxiety, unhealthy anger and symptoms of PTSD.

• Walking tall with swinging arms can help you feel more positive and confident, promoting happiness, according to research. Physical activity is good for any age with innumerable, undeniable health benefits. When one gets older, the goal of exercise is not for speed or quick gain; mobility, balance and stability are the ultimate purposes. There are many forms or patterns of exercise an older individual can safely and comfortably do, and Tai Chi is one of the best mind-body routines to reap wonderful physical and mental benefits. Besides walking, you can try squatting with dumbbells of different weights, pushups with any number of reps tolerable, and band pullaparts.

- Laughter. Smiling and laughing can be the best medicine; it changes your brain's chemistry and makes you feel happier.
- Exercise and break a sweat. It can take as little as five minutes for exercise to put you in a better mood, only if you can physically handle it.
- Practice yoga. Research has shown that it can help promote well-being and improve quality of life in older adults, as well as enhancing senior health with its stress-relieving effects. While some forms of yoga have a spiritual component, yoga can be practiced as a purely physical and physiological exercise, making it compatible with all faith. It is especially ideal for older adults to improve flexibility and fitness, leading to healthy and happy feeling.
- The spiritual life. A spiritual perspective on aging is not just for your own personal transformation; it is a medicine for longevity and health, as shown in many studies. Research shows that people with an active involvement in church or spiritual community are happier and live on average seven years longer than those who don't.

Our body, mind, soul, and spirit are all inter-connected, working synergistically together will give you a life of peace, joy and hope. It is never too late to eat a healthy, balanced diet with 80% fruits and vegetables. Add the supplements of minerals and vitamins when necessary. Do regular physical and brain exercises. Follow the recommended health screenings. Be mindful of personal safety. Have a glass of red wine occasionally or regularly in moderation to reap the health benefits of resveratrol. Do not be afraid to be spiritual.

DR. RICHARD NG, DO

I sincerely pray and hope that you can protect your coming years from potential problems such as the geriatric syndrome of frailty, and keep your golden years shining brightly!

www.ingramcontent.com/pod-product-compliance
Lightning Source LLC
Chambersburg PA
CBHW032055020426
42335CB00011B/354